D0324400

R00196 13705

REF

RA
975.5
.E5
S67   Spencer, James H.
Cop. 1
                      The hospital
                      emergency depart-
                      ment

DATE DUE

DISCARD

REF
RA975.5
.E5
S67   FORM 125M
cop. 1

The Chicago Public Library

MAR 29 1977

Received

The Hospital Emergency Department

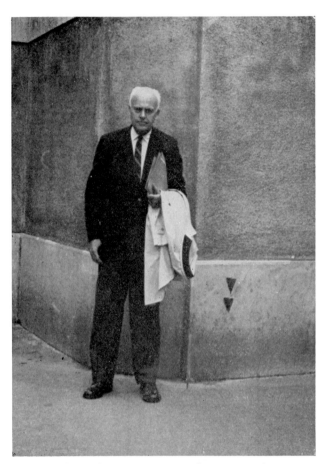

The author at Vienna Accident Hospital.

The Hospital Emergency Department

By

JAMES H. SPENCER, M.D., F.A.C.S.

Medical Director
Morristown Memorial Hospital
Morristown, New Jersey
Former Surgeon-in-Chief
Franklin Hospital
Franklin, New Jersey
Former Chief of Surgery and Chief of Staff
Newton Memorial Hospital
Newton, New Jersey
Former Assistant Director
American College of Surgeons
Secretary
Committee on Trauma
American College of Surgeons

With a Foreword by

ROBERT H. KENNEDY, M.D., F.A.C.S.

Former Director, Field Program
Committee on Trauma
American College of Surgeons

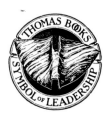

CHARLES C THOMAS • PUBLISHER

Springfield • Illinois • U.S.A.

REF
RA
975.5
.E5
S67
cop. 1

Published and Distributed Throughout the World by
CHARLES C THOMAS • PUBLISHER
BANNERSTONE HOUSE
301–327 East Lawrence Avenue, Springfield, Illinois, U.S.A.

This book is protected by copyright. No part of it may be reproduced in any manner without written permission from the publisher.

© *1972, by* CHARLES C THOMAS • PUBLISHER

ISBN 0–398–02482–0

Library of Congress Catalog Card Number: 71–190337

With THOMAS BOOKS *careful attention is given to all details of manufacturing and design. It is the Publisher's desire to present books that are satisfactory as to their physical qualities and artistic possibilities and appropriate for their particular use.* THOMAS BOOKS *will be true to those laws of quality that assure a good name and good will.*

Printed in the United States of America

BB-14

MAR 2 9 1977

SCI P

To the members of the New Jersey Committee on Trauma of the American College of Surgeons, who took the lead in improvement of Emergency departments in the United States

CONTRIBUTORS

C. H. Hardin Branch, M.D.
Clinical Professor of Psychiatry
University of Southern California
Los Angeles, California
Deputy Director, Mental Health Services
County of Santa Barbara
Santa Barbara, California
Formerly Professor and Chairman
Department of Psychiatry
University of Utah
Salt Lake City, Utah

Richard S. Crampton, M.D.
Associate Professor of Medicine
Director, Mobile and Stable Coronary Care Units
Department of Medicine
University of Virginia Medical Center
Charlottesville, Virginia

William E. Hooper, M.D.
Assistant Professor of Surgery
Director of Emergency Department
Temple University
Philadelphia, Pennsylvania

Chester H. Philips, A.B., M.F.A.
Member, American Institute of Architects
Partner, Epple and Seaman, Architects
Morristown, New Jersey

Arthur F. Southwick, Jr., J.D., M.B.A.
Professor of Business Law
Graduate School of Business Administration
University of Michigan
Ann Arbor, Michigan

Ralph D. Worthylake, M.D.
Clinical Instructor in Psychiatry
University of Oregon Medical School
Portland, Oregon
Psychiatry Staff
Rogue Valley Memorial Hospital
Medford, Oregon

FOREWORD

In each lifetime, change and the adjustment to it are important characteristics. In my own time, spanning nearly three generations, change will possibly appear in history as the most striking feature of the twentieth century. Among other fields, this has been true in the tremendous advances in medical science, in the increased use of hospitals, and in the growing public demand for ready availability and high quality of care. The change in the use of hospital emergency service is a good example.

Within my memory, the accident room in a hospital was a single room to which an ambulatory person might come, or to which an ambulance might bring a nonpaying victim of sudden illness or unexpected trauma. The advent of the motor car, movement of population to our cities, and disappearance of house calls, among other factors, resulted, at least from the period of World War II, in increased use of emergency departments for all types of physical complaints, in all walks of life, at any time of day or night. The accident room became the emergency room, which had to be enlarged and required more personnel around the clock. In some places, more than 100,000 visits a year were made to a facility which grew to forty rooms, with heated arguments as to who should man it. By the late fifties, it came to be recognized that this must be made a hospital department. Papers on the subject of emergency departments began to be presented before medical societies and to appear in the journals, hospital associations and their magazines discussed the subject, hospital trustees and architects became interested.

The problems were found to be legion and to vary with each community. Statistics showed continually an annual increase in patients of about 10 per cent. A million dollars for a new emergency facility was no longer considered a big news item.

Laws began to be passed concerning coverage and personnel. Liability suits against both hospital emergency departments and the doctors manning them became common.

Interest became aroused in national and state governments, in the various national associations concerned, in social and welfare organizations. Strangely enough, although the publications concerning individual items have been legion, there has been no volume covering all aspects of the emergency facility. Dr. James H. Spencer now presents *The Hospital Emergency Department*, as far as I can learn, the first complete volume in this field. I am pleased to have had the opportunity to digest this before its publication. This list of chapter headings shows the breadth of coverage. It lives up to its plan not to include details of treatment. This was a wise decision, for addition of these details would have meant a complete treatise on the practice of medicine—this is available elsewhere. References at the end of many chapters add further value.

Dr. Spencer is eminently fitted to prepare this volume. He is a board-certified general surgeon who throughout his career has had a particular interest in the field of trauma. He was one of the surgical leaders in New Jersey, which was the first state to become interested in emergency department problems, and he continued his interest nationally. In later years, he entered the administrative field and became closely concerned with emergency care from this point of view. He has stressed throughout the variation in required planning according to the details of manner of life and the need in each community. The inordinate waste from lack of preplanning is emphasized. The variance in problems in university, municipal, and community institutions is continually brought to our attention.

Some subjects are in too evolutionary a stage to appear as yet between hard covers. The ultimate place for triage in the philosophy of the emergency department depends on the decision as to the care of the nonemergent patient. Should all general hospitals have emergency departments? This depends in part on what agreement is reached on the practicality and details of categorization of emergency departments. What should be the relationship of the hospital and the emergency department to comprehensive community care? How much responsibility should a hospital take on? More papers, discussion, and symposia are needed before the value and wisdom of these are determined in communities of varying size and character.

This volume is a needed addition to the hospital library and to medical literature. It has been well planned and produced. It should be valuable to hospital trustees, the medical profession, hospital administrators, nurses, architects, and engineers.

New York City ROBERT H. KENNEDY

PREFACE

The emergency department of the general hospital has been the subject of widespread interest in this country for more than two decades. Prior to World War II, this department was frequently housed in a single room even in large hospitals. It was sometimes called the accident room. In hospitals with house staffs, the interns usually took care of the emergencies. They were often not enthusiastic about this assignment, for it did not represent a meaningful learning experience. In hospitals without house staffs, the staffing of the department was a very haphazard affair.

Since World War II, the public has become much more hospital minded. At the same time, doctors have changed their patterns of practice. They are attempting to live more orderly lives. This means more regular hours with a decrease of availability to the public. The sick or injured patient finds it more difficult to get the service of his or any other doctor, whenever he needs them or thinks he does. This has led the public to turn to the hospital for medical care, both emergency and otherwise. Out-patient clinics have not been geared to this influx of more patients, so the only place for the public to go has been the emergency department. This influx caught most hospitals unawares. How they reacted and how they can react are dealt with in various chapters of this book.

One result of this increase in emergency department activity has been a multitude of conferences, speeches, published papers, and other exchanges of ideas on the problems presented I have attended many of these conferences, listened to many of the speeches and made a few of them, and read many of the papers and written a few of them. To my knowledge, no one has yet attempted to bring together between the covers of one book a discussion of the many problems of the emergency department along with discussions of their solutions.

Many books have been written on the treatment of medical and surgical emergencies, but the need has been for a comprehensive discussion of planning, building, equipping, staffing, and administration of the department in which the treatment takes place. When I was asked if I would be willing to bring together a unified discussion of all aspects of emergency department activities, I welcomed the opportunity.

My interest in the subject antidated World War II. It went back to those days when I was literally "on call" for emergencies twenty-hour hours per day in a small hospital with an accident room about eight by twelve feet. In those days, without realizing it at the time, I began to formulate some ideas with regard to the delivery of efficient emergency care. Military experience which followed, of course influenced my thinking. After the war, a series of circumstances led me progressively to devote more effort to emergency planning over and above my primary interest in surgical care of the patient. Association with other physicians with similar thoughts resulted in our attempts to put into action our collective ideas. Fortuitous circumstances led me to the opportunity to study these problems and to participate in planning on a national scale. One thing, however, of which I have become more and more convinced is the need for thoughtful planning at the local level. As pointed out in one of the chapters, national studies are of value, but the problems to be solved are mostly local, and this book is an attempt to help solve them.

As I planned the contents and made an outline I realized that in some areas I lacked both the background and experience to write with authority. From my own knowledge and with the help of friends I selected guest authors for chapters I felt I could not write. Although I have submitted to some of them chapters to show the pattern of the book, I have not influenced them in any way. They have been invited to express their views freely. Each of these guest authors has been selected for precise reasons. They have all had a wealth of experience and have written from that position.

It is my hope that the ideas expressed in this book will be of help to doctors, nurses, administrators, trustees, architects, and hospital consultants as they plan for the ever-increasing and increasingly important problems of the emergency department in the general hospital. I hope it will even be read by those physicians who avoid an appearance in the department, but who use it as a convenient place to send their patients.

If readers sense a somewhat dogmatic attitude in the presentation of some of the ideas, I will be pleased. When I feel secure in my beliefs, I do not hesitate to be dogmatic. I have in many instances presented varying points of view but have tried to defend my own. I ask each reader to consider the theme of the entire work and not to judge it on isolated sections. I also ask him to keep in mind that I firmly believe that emergency departments should be for *emergencies* and that all planning should focus on this belief. This is the viewpoint from which I have written. A weekend in a busy emergency department, where life may hang in the balance and the scales may be tipped by ability or lack of it and by readiness or lack of it, should convince the most skeptical that the emergency department should not be a substitute for the O.P.D. If that statement seems over dramatic, so be it. The emergency department is a dramatic place.

JAMES H. SPENCER

ACKNOWLEDGMENTS

I suppose the genesis of no book could be traced with complete accuracy, certainly not this one. Questions that I have been asked about emergency departments have convinced me that the questioners really wanted help. Those, then, who have asked the questions—doctors, nurses, hospital administrators, trustees, patients, and many others—should first be thanked for focusing the light of inquiry on this complex problem. They could never be enumerated, for they are legion.

However, there are others who have had a direct influence on what has been included in this volume, and the least I can do is thank them publicly. Doctors Roswell K. Brown and J. Cuthbert Owens received early drafts of a number of the chapters, and their suggestions were most valuable. Doctor Robert H. Kennedy was a helpful source of suggestions regarding items to be stressed, and of course I was grateful that a man of his stature willingly wrote the Foreword.

I am indebted to Mrs. Betty Dhandi and Mrs. Beverly Raden, former secretaries in Chicago, for typing early drafts of many of the chapters in their spare time, and to Virginia Fry for "moonlighting" on the final typing. The staff of Charles C Thomas, Publisher, has been most helpful in steering me through the mechanics of publication. Their understanding patience in the presence of a multitude of delays has been comforting.

Finally, my wife, Ruth, has given me in this effort the same encouragement she has always provided. When at times the obstacles to completion seemed insurmountable, she knew just when to encourage me to continue or to forget it until the picture looked brighter. She read and reread draft after draft of most of the chapters and corrected not only syntax but spelling. It is really *our* book, not mine.

J.H.S.

PHOTO CREDITS

CONTENTS

The Hospital Emergency Department

Chapter 1

FUNCTION OF THE EMERGENCY
DEPARTMENT
ITS USE AND MISUSE

"The function of an emergency department is to give adequate appraisal and initial treatment or advice to any person who considers himself acutely ill or injured and presents himself at the emergency department door."

That statement, released after much thought and discussion, is taken directly from the *Standards for Emergency Departments in Hospitals,* formulated by the Committee on Trauma and approved by the Board of Regents of the American College of Surgeons. It would be difficult to define this function more succintly in one sentence.

While in its excellent brochure[1] on emergency departments the American Hospital Association does not present a definition of the function, it does discuss it. This statement is included as follows: "The conclusion is that no patient with a complaint serious enough to bring him to the emergency department of the hospital should be denied appropriate examination and disposition by a physician working with adequate facilities and under appropriate supervision." The brochure further defines the term *emergency department* by saying, "It is intended to signify whatever facilities or services are provided for the management of outpatients coming to the hospital for the treatment of complaints considered to require immediate care in the hospital environment." Again, under the discussion of "Extent and Types of Services" the American Hospital Association warns against the use of the department for "emergency or elective surgical procedures of long duration," because it will affect the availability of facilities and will immobilize person-

3

nel, both of which are needed for the care of other patients. It continues by recommending that inpatient examinations and treatments not be done in the emergency department and concludes with the statement "*It should be used for emergencies only.*"[*]

These statements from responsible organizations interested in this field of health care are straight to the point. There is no reason to interpret them any way but literally. Their interpretation need not allow the public to abuse the facility. No patient coming to the department with a chronic condition that has not taken a turn for the worse can in any reasonable manner consider himself acutely ill. That he should be seen by a physician goes without saying, but that he should necessarily be treated does not. He should have appropriate "examination and disposition"—and the latter may be referral to an appropriate source of treatment. In the selection of this source, he may have a choice if he wishes. Otherwise the choice may be made for him. The opportunity should not be missed to inform him that he has come to the wrong facility for the type of care he requires. Following this policy will help to keep the misuse of the emergency department to a minimum.

The misuse of the emergency department has been noted repeatedly, but it has been interesting to notice the diversity of attitudes toward it. Shortliffe,[2] for instance, reports that "in Great Britain, Canada and the United States, individual studies have all supported the contention that emergency departments have become 'problem areas,' mostly because of the patient loads pressed upon them." He continues, "The studies have also pointed out that the important problem now is not whether the various complaints seen in emergency departments actually constitute emergencies. Rather, the problem is that the public appears to have made its decision to seek out hospital emergency care in times of real or imaginary ailments." Elsewhere, Shortliffe[3] has implied that since the public has made its decision, we must go along with this. With the first statement about "problem areas" we can concur; with the

---

[*]Author's italics.

second we cannot. We believe that something can be done to make the public change its mind. In fact, many hospitals are doing it—examples are given later in this chapter. To adopt the defeatist attitude is to look forward to the time when a hospital will be a department of a huge community health complex centering in the emergency department rather than the reverse.

Reports from England, however, do not seem to support Shortliffe's conclusion.

A study carried out by the Nuffield Provincial Hospitals Trust[4] emphasizes the need for "relieving the hospitals of the burden of such cases," referring to the relatively minor, non-emergent cases. In an editorial, the *Economist*[5] discusses this report under the title "What is a Casualty?" and points out that the Nuffield report notes that the casualty department of a hospital "should be regarded not as a duplicate of a general practitioner's surgery (office) but as a service of urgency and emergency, that is, for injury and sudden illness."

The author has had the opportunity to visit the casualty departments of several British hospitals over the years and to compare their operation with those in this country. One of these, the Radcliffe Infirmary at Oxford, I have visited several times. On the last visit I was told that 75 percent of the patients treated were real emergencies. Inquiring as to how this has been accomplished, I found that the method was the same as that which has proven successful in many American hospitals, education of the public. All patients, I was informed, were seen by a physician who did not hesitate to send some of them home, even without treatment, with instructions to consult their doctors. Of course, this presupposes the availability of doctors.

Shortliffe[6] himself had previously pointed out the fallacy of the "open door" policy in emergency departments when he admitted that "the vast majority of illness can be better and more economically treated in the physician's office and in the home and rightfully in one or the other of these places." Possibly we have misunderstood him when he has mentioned the necessity for enlarging emergency room facilities to take care of an increasing segment of the public that "looks to the hospital in time of need," for he observes, "While it is important that every patient should leave the emergency room feeling that he has been well and completely handled with due consideration for his own personality and individuality, public relations should not lead the emergency room into imperiling its function. Indeed good public relations can never do this. Honesty is necessary at all times and must, on occasion, be accompanied by gentle firmness in rejecting the patient and controlling his overdemonstrative relatives. One should be guided by the rule that the best public relations in the hospital is a good standard of medical and nursing care." If that be true, and it surely is, then the emergency department must be kept ready for real emergencies at all times.

Howell and Buerki[7] also seem to assume that the complete takeover of the hospital emergency unit by the public is inevitable. They say, ". . . it can be anticipated that the number of visits to the emergency unit will increase, particularly at odd hours of the day." They continue, "This would indicate then that the traditional emergency room, often only a temporary medical haven for free service, will soon disappear. In its stead will emerge the future emergency unit designed for total medical care, melding together *some* of the features of true emergency service with those of extensive outpatient diagnosis and treatment."[*]

Then, after indicating that this huge complex will have only "some of the features of true emergency service," they go on to say that the department should be ready for all emergencies at all hours. "All medical personnel should be schooled in emergency diagnosis and treatment; each should be completely familiar with procedures and equipment; each should be on hand to fulfill his role in the emergency team." That is a large order for everyone assigned to this complex majoring in "extensive outpatient diagnosis and treatment." If true emergency care is to be salvaged from this extensive plan, the author believes it will have to move to new quarters!

The health advisors to President Lyndon Johnson had so

[*] Author's italics.

convinced him of the overuse of hospital emergency rooms that he included this among the major health problems confronting the United States in his Health Message[8] to Congress in 1967.

The emergency department deserves departmental status in the table of organization of the hospital, but only if its main and almost exclusive function is care of emergencies. If it spreads itself into "extensive outpatient diagnosis and treatment," it becomes only an outpatient clinic. This is not an orderly, well-organized clinic, with specialists doing the diagnosis and treatment, but a catch-as-catch-can affair with ample opportunities for serious errors of omission. With patients having all kinds of chronic conditions—some of them serious— coming to the emergency department at all hours, the harassed emergency room doctor, knowing that these are not emergencies, may give slighting attention to them in order that he may be free to devote his attention to those who need him immediately.

These nonemergency patients are the ones that Shortliffe states can be better and more economically treated in the physician's office and in the home. Would it not be a service to them to direct them to the facility where they will get better care and save money? This process of education against misuse, this propaganda if you insist, is surely in the public interest. The next day, the patient who shouldn't have been there may be back with a real emergency, and he will be the gainer if the way is cleared for prompt attention. The patient who should be educated out of the emergency department is the one Duncan[9] refers to as the one "who uses the emergency room for his personal convenience." She reports that at the 900-bed Methodist Hospital in Indianapolis, a study of 3000 consecutive emergency-room patients showed 49 percent to be accidental injuries. Of the remainder, about 8 percent of the total were also emergencies or urgent. Twenty-one percent were "less urgent" but still needing prompt attention. The remaining 22 percent were those who "use the emergency room for their personal convenience." This percentage is better than in some other large general hospitals in big cities.

In discussing what an emergency is, Davidson[10] states, "Experience seems to force us to define an emergency as any condition in a patient considered in urgent need of medical care by the patient, his family, friends, the police department, or whoever assumes the responsibility for bringing the patient to the hospital." He quite rightly concludes that these people should have medical care. He continues however, "There is another large group of patients who tend to use the emergency room who do not fall within this definition." He adds, "There is an increasing demand on both private and city and charity hospitals to perform an additional function which is becoming a *stifling** burden. Many indigent patients, as well as private patients, expect the emergency service to function as a 24-hour doctor's office or clinic for their non-emergency problems. . . . The community should be educated by whatever means possible to recognize that the emergency service is for patients who feel they have an acute, urgent medical need, and that it is not an economical or convenient doctor's office or clinic."

"An emergency area and its staff cannot be enlarged rapidly enough to keep up with the growing popularity of its service, should it encourage such patients to seek help there." Davidson feels that in the case of these people who must be taken care of, "the answer to this problem is to expand the outpatient department to absorb this additional load, instead of cluttering the emergency area or confusing the management of emergency cases in the emergency area."

This is the voice of reason. An emergency department that is "cluttered" with people not needing emergency care cannot fulfill its responsibility to the community. In contrast to Davidson's advice to enlarge other facilities, it is interesting to note that another large hospital of the same general type enlarged its emergency department three times. This is one of the hospitals, which by its own admission, has let the public establish its policies.

The implementation of Titles 18 and 19 of the Social Security legislation has had an impact on the emergency department

* Author's italics.

situation. Passage of a law does not increase the number of medical or surgical emergencies, but in some places it has created an emergency situation in departments not prepared for an increase in applicants for all kinds of medical care. People in the age and economic groups eligible for the benefits of this legislation are likely to be ones who will seek all kinds of medical care through other-than-private channels. A quasi-beneficent government, while claiming to solve the medical problems of its dependents, has in reality compounded these and other problems in the case of the provident ones who by planning and foresight have prepared for such eventualities. Savings that would have provided for medical care and other needs have been diluted to the extent that they are inadequate for such needs. Inflation, brought on in no small degree by government planning far beyond that which might have been required, has made medical paupers of prideful people who would have much preferred to care for themselves. By not limiting these expenditures to a plan aimed only at the needy, government has wasted millions on those who do not need this help. The wealthy benefit by it, going to the hospital and occupying the same private rooms they would have used anyway, but paying only the difference between the government handout and the total bill. The poor still go to the lesser quarters, and so do not escape the "means test" so decried by the federal government spokesmen making promises that can only be kept with other peoples' resources. Regardless of political party in power, there is every reason to believe that government financing of medical care will continue to spread until it covers a large segment of the population. It could only be stopped by a major change in both executive and legislative philosophy. The present mood of the American electorate is to depend more and more on federal government support, so it is unlikely that enough men can be put in office and kept there long enough to stem the tide of overall socialism. That being the case, hospitals must prepare to care for everyone for everything whenever they want it, if they expect to get even a portion of what is rightfully due them from federal funds drained from or squeezed out of the local collective coffers. It is not a bright picture because, politicians to the contrary, there will be more and more in the way of "standards" set up in Washington. Only the naive fail to recognize these as veiled government controls, a thing we have been promised we would not have.

Hospital planners at the local level who have the interests of the sick and injured at heart must face this situation. If they hope to provide capable emergency services, they must devise means of divorcing these services from those to be provided to the waves of government-encouraged and government-financed patients who will overrun these institutions demanding everything from preventive medicine to intensive care on their own terms. One of the most practical solutions is the physical and administrative separation of emergency services from all others. Halfway measures will produce halfway results. Some hospitals have already demonstrated this.

THE HOSPITAL'S RESPONSIBILITY

All hospitals, regardless of their type, owe certain responsibilities to the public. The general hospital, when it opens its doors, may reasonably be expected to offer to the public a variety of facilities, some of which may not be found in a hospital known to devote its program to a limited field of health care. One of these is an emergency department. A hospital functioning solely for the care of chronic chest diseases, obstetrics, or some other limited medical program need not provide facilities for the care of medical or surgical emergencies in other fields, but the community has a right to expect that the general hospital will.

That the public, while rightfully expecting such care, has in some instances interfered with its quality is a fact that needs to be understood. The situation is a complex one, but the misuse of emergency departments in general hospitals has become a major concern of many responsible people in hospital circles. That the public shares in the guilt and has acted contrary to its own interests is self-evident, but only an enlightened public may be expected to mend its ways. A process of prophylactic education might have helped to prevent the situation in which many hospitals now find themselves, but it is too late for that.

The fact is that the emergency departments of too many hospitals have deteriorated into round-the-clock general medical clinics, and in doing so have become less able to fulfill their real function.

Little help can be offered to physicians and administrators who have surrendered to the misuse concept as an inevitable trend of the times. Fortunately many have not. This group includes some who have lost the first battle but refuse to surrender. They have come to believe, or have always believed, that a literal definition should be applied to the term *emergency department,* and they hope to stem the tide and reverse the trend. Some of this group have confessed that they have been caught unaware and have recorded their efforts to undo the damage. Their experiences should prove profitable to fellow sufferers, but only if the corrective measures are noted. Any hospital may attempt a correction of this situation with reasonable hope of success if all the forces are mustered and defeatism abandoned.

It cannot be repeated too often that any reform, any corrective program in emergency department abuse, must be the joint effort of the hospital administration, medical staff, and the community. Any unilateral effort is doomed to failure.

The American Hospital Association[1] has expressed this well: "The emergency department should be regarded as a distinct and valuable community resource, the responsibility for which is shared between the hospital as a community institution and the medical profession. This approach makes it possible to conduct an effective community education program, designed to limit abuse and secure optimum utilization of all available emergency care facilities. Aware of these facts and conscious of their obligation, medical staffs and administrators of hospitals are faced with the responsibility of examining the problem from the point of view of the individual institution."

WHAT HAS HAPPENED IN YOUR HOSPITAL?

The accumulation of state or nationwide statistics has its value, but sometimes they seem to be collected to prove something that is self-evident. If Kennedy's indictments of Emergency Departments in 1954 and many times since be true, and they surely are, then what we need is a maximum effort to improve conditions.

If statistics are collected with a long-range plan to repeat the study several years later, following efforts toward improvement, they have value. However, with the limited manpower available, it would seem appropriate to devote the major effort to making things better rather than to telling how bad they are. An analogy may be drawn with one of the chief statistics-collecting organizations connected with the practice of medicine, the Commission on Professional and Hospital Activities. The program of this agency is the collection of statistics having to do with quality of patient care in hospitals, yet seldom does it publish anything indicating how good or bad the overall picture is. Dr. Virgil Slee, the Director, has said, "Our chief function is service to the individual hospital, not collecting national statistics." His approach to the improvement of care in hospitals compares favorably with the approach of Curry to improvement of transportation of the injured. The author[11] has shown that Curry was more concerned with pointing out local deficiencies to those responsible than he was with publishing the whole dismal picture. More on this philosophy will be found in Chapter 19, "Evaluation—Emergency Department Surveys."

The facts important to each hospital are not "national trends," "changing patterns," or any of the other catchy phrases that have been coined to cover up the fact that hospitals have been caught off guard. Don't look upstate or across the river or out West to see what is happening. Look in the mirror. What has happened to you? Knowing about someone else's troubles won't help. Try to figure out what you did wrong. Why did the public take over? Were your doctors not available in their offices or to make calls? Have they been referring their weekend calls to the hospital? If so, find out if they are willing to help solve the problem.

Did you encourage this flooding of the emergency department in order to advertise your facilities? Were you using the emergency department as a "loss leader"? If so, do you wish you hadn't? Did you miss the opportunity to educate the public about the real purpose, and what is more important, the real value of the department?

When you have asked these questions and gotten the answers, you will be in a position to try to get out of trouble. Don't take comfort in fellow sufferers, but do try to find out what they are doing to solve this problem. Look at the hospitals where the problem isn't acute and see what they did to prevent it. There are lots of them. Look at the hospitals that have the problem but are trying to solve it. Look at Yale–New Haven and its triage system.

This large hospital of over 700 beds is affiliated with Yale University School of Medicine and has a complete complement of interns and residents. Located as it is in an area (to quote its spokesmen) ". . . of economically independent, socially isolated, minority population groups, who are often recent arrivals to these old communities and have only remote connections to the 'usual' pattern of private medical care," it has felt the changes in emergency department patterns. Weinerman and Edwards,[12] in recounting the Yale–New Haven experience, say, "The role of the general hospital has changed from that of a last resort for the seriously ill to a community resource for a broad spectrum of general medical care services to ambulatory patients." They continue, "The resulting use in the volume, and particularly, in the requirements of care for the non-urgent, often complex and chronic disorders, have taxed the resources and the systems of most emergency facilities. The impacts are felt in terms of inadequacy of space and layout, of equipment and staff, of procedures and finances. The relationships of hospitals with professional groups and the community at large undergo increasing strain. As usual, the administrator gets the blame, and the private inpatient pays the bill." Probably no statement has summed up all facets of this problem so tersely as this.

Finding themselves in this predicament, those responsible at Yale–New Haven considered the available alternatives and determined on a "triage" system, which they refer to as "initial evaluation and selected referral of all entering emergency service patients." The detailed report of their plan and its results is well-worth reading, but may be summarized as follows:

1. Immediate assignment for emergency attention within the emergency service.
2. Short wait in turn for less urgent care, also within the emergency service.
3. Referral for immediate or subsequent care to an outpatient clinic or private office.
4. Referral to another community agency.
5. Direct discharge.

If the condition is a minor one and the treatment simple, the whole matter may be completed by the triage officer.

At the time of reporting, the statement was made that the system seemed to have improved the quality and convenience of service to patients, eased the administrative burden, and improved community relationships. In addition to this qualitative evaluation, the quantitative result has been significant. The steady uptrend in visits has been slowed. While the visits in the year before this triage system was instituted had been 8.1 percent higher than the previous year, the new system had reduced the visits slightly. The qualitative improvement is just as important as the quantitative slackening. Both can do nothing but improve sound public relations.

In a more recent report from Yale–New Haven, Beloff[13] indicates that the good results of the triage system have continued. While the number of patients going to the emergency department over a three-year period had increased, the rate of increase was slowed, and there was a decrease in percentage of medical cases by the end of this period. Probably the best result was the increase in percentage of patients that were dealt with through other than the true emergency service— in other words, channeled off to the facilities to which better judgment would have directed them in the first place. One of the by-products of this was, according to Beloff, ". . . to allow more time for the medical and surgical residents to treat the serious major emergencies."

No doubt there have been disgruntled patients at Yale–New

Haven, but judging from the reports by several authors, this has been a minor factor. Persistent adherence to a carefully conceived plan continues to pay dividends in New Haven over a long period.

There would be fewer patients to triage in the situation just described if the nonemergency patients could be routinely directed through another entrance. In a recent (1970) visit to St. Bartholomew's Hospital in London, the author found a newly constructed outpatient department wisely planned. The facilities for emergencies were separate from those for the nonemergent clinic patients. The entrances were also separate for the two classes of patients. It was obvious that the planners had given serious thought to keeping nonemergencies out of the "casualty department." This is at least a partial solution to a long-existing problem at St. Bartholomew's, as will be noted later in this chapter.

Another hospital that has approached this problem in a different way is Ingalls Memorial Hospital at Harvey, Illinois.[14] A publicity campaign was launched to "make these facilities more fully available for legitimate emergencies, while maintaining and reinforcing the community's knowledge that the hospital stands ready at all times to provide top quality professional services for the sick and injured." Local newspapers explained to the public the true purpose of the emergency department and urged the public to "get in touch with your family physician first." Twenty thousand leaflets paid for by the medical staff were distributed in doctors' offices, bus and railway stations, and banks. These leaflets explained that the emergency room is not a substitute for the doctor's office. This paid off. Although in this rapidly growing community the emergency case load continued to increase, the rate of increase diminished. The important result was that the percentage of unwarranted cases decreased. The report continues, "Based on present indications, it is felt that the hospital will continue to experience relief from emergency service misuse. Thousands of families have been reached by the program who have not as yet been faced with a situation they might otherwise have viewed as warranting a trip to the hospital emergency room.

"Staff physicians report that many families are now calling them first rather than coming directly to the hospital emergency room. They are thus able to avert many more unnecessary trips than formerly. Doctors have also reported that many families, other than newcomers, have visited their offices to get acquainted before they have need of medical services."

A campaign such as this to decrease the use of emergency departments for nonemergencies will highlight the real purpose of the department and thus probably increase the overall use. This is good, for it is increasing the value of the department to the community. The campaign is not one to avoid work but to make the work most worthwhile.

Actually, in some reports there have been exaggerations about the use of these departments for nonemergencies. So many statistics regarding the classification of patients coming to emergency departments have been published that the whole matter becomes confusing. Some conclusions have been drawn that do not indicate a very sophisticated analysis of the statistics. For instance, statements that imply that patients with medical, obstetrical, or pediatric problems are not emergencies are not sound. While it is true that a majority of emergencies are surgical, particularly the results of injury, there are other acute emergencies. Some of these demand as good judgment and as prompt action as the traumatic injuries. These are stressed in the chapters on medical and psychiatric emergencies.

As has been mentioned, this problem of overuse of emergency departments is not limited to the United States. Neither is it just a recent phenomenon. A report in the *Lancet* 100 years ago describes the rapid increase in numbers of patients coming to St. Bartholomew's Hospital outpatient department. It was the casualty patients causing most of the increase. Again in 1910, a report of King Edward's Hospital Fund Committee notes, "It is said that there is a tendency for the casualty department to grow until it becomes a duplicate outpatient department, differing from the outpatient department proper in being subject to less regulation as regards hours of attendance and inquiry into circumstances. True casualties, however, if

their numbers were recorded, would stand in a class by themselves. . . . They would comprise injuries by accident and
sudden attacks of illness which require immediate attention
and treatment."

Here we detect the British patients of pre-World War I
times coming at hours "for their personal convenience" and
bypassing the social service office; an example of the fact that
we learn from the British if given enough time!

We also find that some of the measures we are taking today
to lessen the burden in emergency departments were in use in
England long before. In 1932, another King's Fund Committee
mentions that in some hospitals, the casualty officers who are
resident or junior medical officers are empowered to send
minor cases away to a private doctor or to some other agency
after one examination or treatment.

The Nuffield report[4] sheds some light on the effectiveness
of efforts to keep down the load in casualty departments. In
17 hospitals with an average annual number of casualty department visits of 19,600 each in 1958, the nontraumatic or
nonurgent cases were kept down to 12 percent. The control
methods may be described as just plain courteous public education. They were as follows:

1. Polite notice, backed up by informing general practitioners of the function of the department and asking for
   their cooperation, as well as "friendly persuasion" by the
   staff.
2. No attempt at a barrier on the part of the H.M.C. or consultant staff in a formal way, but polite dissuasion by the
   casualty officer and nursing staff.
3. Rigid barrier notice, without explanation, blacklisting de-
   faulting general practitioners, turning patients back without seeing a casualty officer.
4. Complete open door policy, encouraging patients to use
   casualty as an alternative general practitioner's service,
   with a high ratio of return treatments.
5. Absolutely no attempt at regulation although complaining
   about the overload of trivial cases.

Depending on the measures taken, the percentages of non-emergencies varied from nil to 30 percent, the higher percentages being where policies 4 and 5 were followed. In only one instance were the results not consistent with the efforts made. This is pretty conclusive evidence that the job can be done with English-speaking people!

It is in such places as Yale–New Haven, Ingalls Memorial, and these English hospitals that effective leadership has been demonstrated in curbing the misuse of emergency departments. It is in such places that you will receive help—not in reading statistics showing that only a minority of patients coming to emergency departments have emergencies.

If the study done by Skudder, McCarroll, and Wade[15] in 265 widely scattered hospitals can be taken as a fair sampling, most of the people involved want to limit the department to caring for emergencies. Three-fourths of the hospitals replied that "the function of an emergency department should be restricted to the care of patients with actual emergency conditions." One-half claimed that they could do this. Even this firmly rebuts the claim that all varieties of cases *must* be treated if the public demands it. Assuming that the one-fourth of these hospitals which do not believe that the department should be for emergencies only make no effort to limit attendance, it is clear that two-thirds of those trying have succeeded. The remaining third may be encouraged by the fact they are in the minority.

Correcting abuse will not be easy. The suggestion that unnecessary visits can be curbed is only for those in favor of it. Where the medical staff, administrator and trustees truly feel that the department best serves the community when operated as an around-the-clock outpatient department, this is the policy that should be followed. If "changing patterns" is what you want, then so be it.

If a change is proposed, it should be based strictly on local needs and desires, not on national trends. National trends have led many people and many groups into trouble in many walks of life. A veritable council of war is called for, and representatives of medical staff, administration, trustees, nursing department, and even the public should participate. A substantial majority of these must be in agreement with the aims to be accomplished. It must be recognized that there will be dissenters, but if they are in the minority, patient pressure should be brought to bear on them. The roots of the evil must be removed and this will require some soul-searching, particularly among medical staff and administration.

WHO IS AT FAULT?

The answer must be sought to the question, "Was necessity back of the trend of the public to bypass doctor's offices and established clinics with regular hours?" If the doctors have not been available to care for nonemergencies in facilities outside the emergency departments, they must confess it, and this confessional must not be limited to the generalist. There are entirely too many medical specialists who have become so independent that the patient is made to feel he is receiving a favor when he is treated. If American doctors truly believe in and want "free enterprise" in medicine and want the spirit of competition, they must be enterprising. Playing hard to-get will not help their cause.

It is pretty difficult to justify a complete absence of evening or weekend office hours by specialists in a community where some patients can't get to a doctor's office in the daytime. To contend that such inconvience as evening office hours should only be suffered by general practitioners is to downgrade the general practitioner. One of the reasons general practice has become unpopular is this downgrading and lack of status, and one of the reasons some general practitioners try to gain status and escape their fate by delving into fields in which they are not trained is the unwillingness of specialists to share in the inconveniences inherent in the care of patients. Is there any reason why such specialists as the general surgeon, the orthopedist, and the obstetrician, to name three, should not be available for evening appointments at least once a week? Their presence in their offices on Saturday mornings would be a boon to many busy, hard-working patients.

If it could be known that doctors were going to be available at hours convenient to the public, one of the big steps toward clearing the emergency rooms of nonemergencies would be taken. It is not stretching the theory of hospital staff responsibility to expect this. After all, it is simply a united effort to solve a pressing community and hospital problem. Horrified as some of them may be, the city specialists need feel no immunity to their responsibility. After all, these are "changing times" in which we live.

CAN ADMINISTRATION HELP?

Does the outpatient department program need review? Does it need explaining to the public? Has the fact that it can offer better care of nonemergent conditions been stressed in publicity? Would a physical facility in the hospital, divorced from the emergency department, in which staff doctors may see private patients by appointments, relieve some of the pressure? This is nothing new. It will be discussed in another chapter.

A rereading of the definition of an emergency department and a reappraisal of the situation in each hospital could change the whole trend. It might establish a "pattern" from which everyone would benefit.

I .

REFERENCES

1. *The Emergency Department in the Hospital: A Guide to Organization and Management.* Chicago, American Hospital Association, 1962.
2. Shortliffe, E.C.: The emergency department: some considerations on essential physical facilities. *Hospitals, 36*:48–50, 1962.
3. Shortliffe, E.C., Hamilton, T.S., and Noroian, E.H.: The emergency room and the changing pattern of medical care. *N Eng J Med, 258*:20–25, 1958.
4. *Casualty Services and Their Setting.* London, Oxford University Press, 1960.
5. What is a casualty? *Economist,* Sept. 24, 1960.
6. Shortliffe, E.C.: *Hospitals, 34*:32–34, 1960.
7. Howell, J.T., and Buerki, R.C.: *Hospitals, 31*:37–49, 1957.
8. *Bull of the Assoc Am Med Colleges, Vol.* 2(3):2, 1967.
9. Duncan, Margaret: How to evaluate emergency room care. *Mod Hosp., 99*:103–6, 1962.

10. Davidson, R.A.: *Hospital Topics*, Feb. 1963.

11. Spencer, J.H.: Subcommittee on transportation of the injured. In Curry, G.J.: *Immediate Care and Transport of the Injured.* Springfield, Thomas, 1965.

12. Weinerman, E.R., and Edwards, H.R.: Triage system shows promise in management of emergency department load. *Hospitals,* 38:55–62, 1964.

13. Beloff, J.S.: Adopting the hospital emergency service organization to patient needs. *Hospitals, 42*:8, 1968.

14. Ingalls Memorial Hospital emergency service educational program. *Public Relations News Letter. American Hospital Association,* 1962.

15. Skudder, P.A., McCarroll, J.R., and Wade, P.A.: Hospital emergency facilities and services—A survey. *Bull Am Coll Surgeons, 46*:44–50, 1961.

Chapter 2

LOCATION AND ENTRANCE

There are many hospital architects whose advice in planning the construction of an emergency department would be valuable, but caution should be exercised in letting them make the original suggestions. They should first be well indoctrinated by a committee made up largely of people who are to be responsible for patient care in the department. The time will come when the architect will not only be helpful, but his services will be essential. If he attends committee meetings and becomes imbued with the thought that what is being planned is a service, with the physical structure subordinate to this, he will save much of his time and that of the committee.

There is no better way to begin the planning than to think in terms of a severely injured patient being brought to the hospital by strangers to the community. They naturally expect to find the hospital easily and then the emergency department, and they expect that from the moment of their arrival, all activities will center around prompt and efficient patient care in a proper environment.

DIRECTIONAL SIGNS

Such thinking suggests hospital directional signs on highways, a plainly marked sign at the entrance to the hospital grounds, and directions to the emergency department clearly visible, day or night.

The road signs will, of course, be planned and located under the authority of the responsible highway department, whether it be town, county, or state. They should be so placed as to be foolproof to strangers. Too often road signs of various kinds are put up by local people who take for granted some knowledge of the community.

The signs on the hospital property may be planned entirely by hospital authority. The most important feature is visibility. Several years ago, Doctor Robert H. Kennedy and the author were surveying the emergency department of a hospital and, in the course of our questioning, we asked about a directional sign. "Oh, didn't you see the big sign with an arrow on the corner of the building?" we were asked. A quick trip outside revealed that growing shrubbery had almost obscured what had once been a most adequate marker. Owens[1] found that 13 of 72 hospitals in Colorado had no sign denoting the emergency entrance. Only eight of the 72 had their emergency department signs lighted.

LOCATION

Here there are no choices. The emergency department should be on the ground floor, not up on the fifth floor "to be near x-ray" where it was found in one Pennsylvania hospital. This is not an isolated instance. Skudder, McCarroll, and Wade[2] report that 37 out of 265 hospitals had emergency departments not accessible from the street. This would suggest the old habit of putting this department where no other department wanted to be.

It should not only be on the ground floor, but should have an outside entrance leading directly into the department. Long passageways or circuitous routes through or past other departments risk blockage that may delay immediate care of patients. It is well to locate it in close proximity to the laboratory and x-ray departments. Many of the true emergency-type patients need these departments to aid in their diagnosis. In large hospitals, where the emergency department is a complete self-supporting unit, facilities for x-ray and laboratory studies may be incorporated in it. In most hospitals, this will not be the case. Planning the department near these supporting facilities will prove most worthwhile. If these departments are far removed from each other, it is more important to have the emergency facility close to x-ray. In the case of the laboratory, the technician usually comes to the patient. When x-rays are to be taken, the patient is usually transmitted to the equipment.

Barry[3] states that in a study of 60,000 emergency visits, 30 percent of the patients needed x-ray studies, and Weinerman and Edwards[4] report that 24 percent needed x-rays at Grace–New Haven Hospital.

ENTRANCE

The entrance includes the outside area immediately adjacent to the door or doors, as well as the doors themselves. Whether the entrance is approached by a driveway or not, thought should be given to easy ingress and egress of ambulances and other vehicles. Room for ambulances to turn before or after unloading should be planned in a way not to interfere with others following. This is of extreme importance in the event of a catastrophe resulting in many vehicles coming in. Some of these may have drivers unacquainted with the hospital.

This area may be a wide paved space as shown in the accompanying photographs taken at the Chilton Memorial Hospital, Pompton Plains, New Jersey (Fig. 1) and at the University of West Virginia Hospital, Morgantown, West Virginia (Fig. 2). Another good arrangement is a circular driveway at the end of an approach lane, with ambulances going counterclockwise around the circle, unloading and leaving without having to back into the doorway. Probably the most efficient arrangement is that seen at the Harrisburg (Pennsylvania) Hospital (Fig. 3) and at the Radcliffe Infirmary, Oxford, England (Figs. 4 and 5). Here ambulances enter a driveway from one street, unload at the entrance and continue in the same direction out to another street. This eliminates any possibility of a bottleneck, even though a whole convoy of vehicles may be bringing in patients.

The best planned approaches may be rendered inefficient if a *No Parking* rule is not enforced. *No Parking* signs are not enough, as illustrated by the situation in one of the accompanying photos (Fig. 3). Staff members and hospital employees must not be allowed to leave their cars at the entrance "just for a minute." People in private cars bringing sick or injured

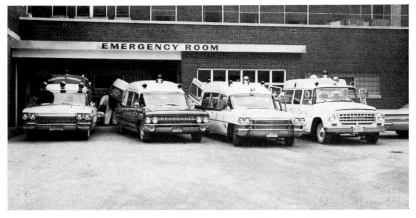

Figure 1. Ambulance entrance, Chilton Memorial Hospital, Pompton Plains, New Jersey.

patients to the emergency department naturally want to go in with their friends or relatives. Someone must courteously, but firmly, direct them to move their car to a designated parking area, or a hospital employee must do it for them. Needless to say, such an area must be provided nearby. These are minor details but may have major significance in an emergency.

Entrances may be of several types. While doors opening out are important in hospitals and may well be required by fire

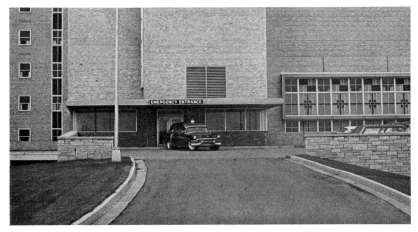

Figure 2. Ambulance entrance, University of West Virginia Hospital, Morgantown, West Virginia.

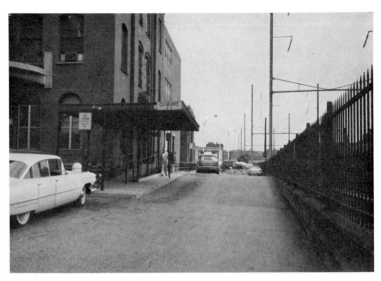

Figure 3. Ambulance entrance, Harrisburg Hospital, Harrisburg, Pennsylvania. This is the drive-through type.

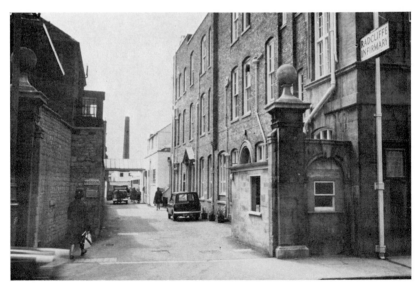

Figure 4. Ambulance entrance, Radcliffe Infirmary, Oxford, England. This is the drive-through type.

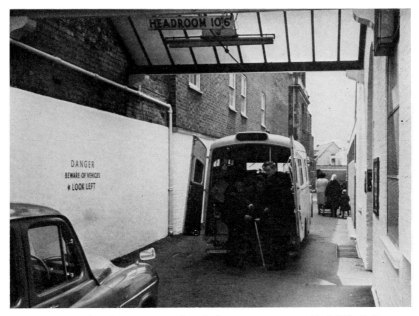

Figure 5. Overhead protection of ambulance entrance at Radcliffe Infirmary.

regulations, it must be remembered that in an emergency department there is more often a need to enter than to exit in a hurry. This suggests a two-way swinging door. Whether the door is single or double is not so important as its width. It should be wide enough to allow attendants to walk on either side of a litter or stretcher as it is taken in. The two-way entrance and exit at the emergency department of the John Gaston Memorial Hospital, Memphis, Tennessee (Fig. 6) is very good as it allows easy ingress and egress with no likelihood of competing traffic. It would be even better if the doors were wider. These doors open automatically by means of an electric treadle.

Protection from the elements should be considered in entrance construction. An overhanging roof or canopy as seen in the illustrations of the Chilton and West Virginia Hospitals is ideal (Figs. 7 and 2). In both of these, it may be seen that a patient may be removed from the rear end of an ambulance without being exposed to rain or snow. The same feature applied to the drive-through type of entrance may be seen in

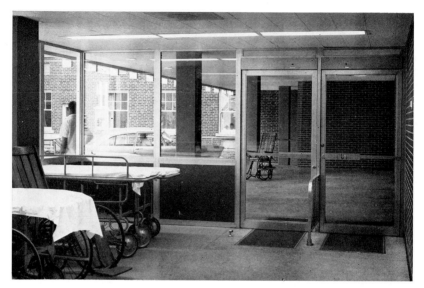

Figure 6. Emergency department entrance, John Gaston Memorial Hospital, University of Tennessee, Memphis, Tennessee. This shows overhead protection, automatic doors, and good stretcher and wheelchair storage.

Figure 5 at the Radcliffe Infirmary. As this entrance is also used for ambulatory patients going to and from the emergency department, a sign is posted to warn them of vehicular traffic.

A CURB OR NOT

Opinions vary with respect to the area onto which stretchers are unloaded. Some maintain that there should be no elevation, while many hospitals have a curb six inches or more in height. Where ambulances back in, this prevents them from going too far. If a curb is constructed, it should be painted white or bright yellow to attract attention, so that no one will trip over it. Another arrangement is to have it about the height of the floor of an ambulance so that ambulance stretchers may be rolled out onto it. This is the type of construction described by Maffly[5] and Jackson at the Herrick Memorial Hospital, Berkeley, California (Fig. 8). This is really a dock, not a curb. When constructed, there should be steps or, better, a ramp to one side as shown here. This would allow easy en-

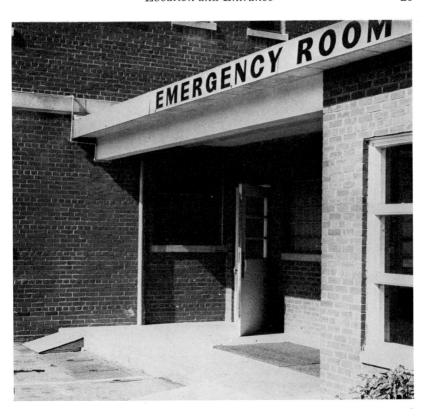

Figure 7. Overhead protection of ambulance entrance at Chilton Memorial Hospital, Pompton Plains, New Jersey.

trance of ambulatory patients and wheel chairs. This illustration also shows good entrance lighting.

CONSTRUCTION

Floor construction in emergency departments is discussed elsewhere, but it is appropriate to mention here that a slip-proof floor is particularly desirable at the entrance. Patients and attendants will come in with wet shoes and in the winter with snow caked on their heels. A corrugated floor or rubber matting may prevent further accidents. If the rubber matting is thick, it may be recessed to floor level to prevent tripping on the edges.

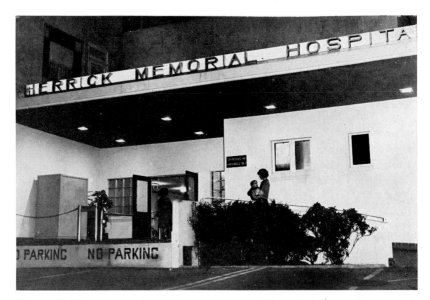

Figure 8. Emergency department entrance, Herrick Memorial Hospital, Berkeley, California. This shows the dock-type of ambulance entrance and a ramp for ambulatory and wheelchair patients. The night picture shows good lighting.

Of four patients operated on by the author in one month because of fracture of the neck of the femur, two were injured at the hospital—one from a fall at the emergency room entrance.

Unless the department is so staffed that any patient coming through the entrance will be seen immediately, some type of signal, such as a buzzer, is useful. This is seldom needed in daylight hours, but at night particularly in small hospitals it serves to alert the personnel on duty that a patient has arrived.

Detailed discussion, with floor plans of emergency room layout, will be found in the following chapter, but it may be well to mention here that a nurses' station with full view of the entrance should be included in any plans for new construction. The charge nurse responsible for patient care, whether she be one of a full staff or working alone at night in a small department, should be able to form a quick opinion of the situation,

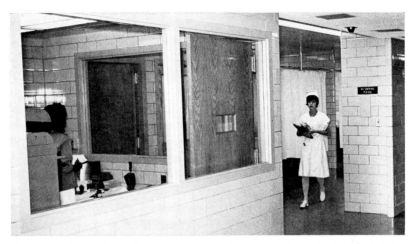

Figure 9. Nurses' station, emergency department, University of West Virginia Hospital. Both the entrance and the working area may be seen through large windows.

so that she may be guided as to what additional personnel she may wish to call. Having the nurses' station glassed-in has many advantages, including protection from drafts in cold weather. Such a nurses' station at the University of West Virginia Hospital is shown in Figure 9. Here the entering patient passes directly in front of the large glass window of the nurses' station, and another window provides a full view of the treatment area.

REFERENCES

1. Owens, J.C.: Travelers need signs locating hospital care. *Mod Hosp*, *106*:95–98, 1966.
2. Skudder, P.A., McCarroll, J.R., and Wade, P.A.: Hospital emergency facilities and services: A survey. *Bull Am Coll Surgeons*, *46*:44–50, 1961.
3. Barry, R.N., Shortliffe, E.C., and Wetston, H.J.: *Hospitals*, *34*:23, 1960.
4. Weinerman, E.R., and Edwards, H.R.: *Hospitals*, *38*, 1964.
5. Maffly, A.E., and Jackson, H.X.: *Mod Hosp.*, *73*:6, pp. 54–58.

Chapter 3

PLANS AND PLANNING

THE COMMITTEE

To assure that a hospital emergency department will best serve the community, it should not be planned hurriedly. The initial planning should be entrusted to a carefully selected committee. Such a committee should have, as a minimum, representation from the medical staff, nursing service, hospital administration, and board of trustees. Naturally, the services of an architect will be needed before much preliminary work is done. Consultation with others will be valuable from time to time. This may even include responsible representation from the public. The committee making the original plans may not be the same as the one to supervise the department after it begins to function, but there may be some who will remain in order to assure continuity of philosophy.

All selections must be carefully made. This is a working committee, not an honorary one. Doctors and nurses chosen should not be appointed because of staff positions held, but on the basis of demonstrated interest and knowledge. Unless a doctor is willing to give unstintingly of his time, his services will be of limited value. Doctors should be appointed with the full knowledge and, if possible, approval of the medical staff. This will minimize the amount of post-construction criticism by the staff. They will be well advised to take proposals back to the staff regarding construction, if there be any possibility of differences of opinion. It must be recognized that most medical staffs have one or two members who will object to anything, unless they propose it in the first place. The author has seen this delay much-needed construction on more than one occasion. Taking ideas back to the staff is a calculated risk, but one that must be taken. The obstructionists will usually make the most use of the improved facilities after they are built.

A nurse to serve on this committee must also be one who shows an interest in the type of work to be done. She need not be the chief nurse of the hospital but should work closely with that individual.

Administration should not only be represented but should have a major voice in decisions. Trustee representation goes without saying, for this body must approve the plans and provide the funds. Whether to look for a trustee in the building trades is a moot question. A public-spirited citizen interested in the best possible emergency service will be a wise choice.

To be determined first is the type of service to be provided for and, after this, the construction and equipment to provide such service. Don't make the mistake of planning the construction first and then fitting the program to it. If the hospital is not a new one and has in the past provided an emergency service, a record of the department's activities and trends should be studied. Any attempt to alter these trends should be considered now, for there will be no better opportunity to change the emergency department philosophy.

Among the features that should influence planning are the following:

1. Rate of growth of population of the community.
2. Predictable changes in the community.
    a. If in a city, is the neighborhood changing? Is the percentage of medically indigent patients increasing or decreasing?
    b. Is it becoming more industrialized, and are the industries of the type that will produce more accidents? (Chemical plants, machine shops, and foundries are more likely to be accident producers than textile mills and publishing houses.)
3. Highway planning, particluarly of heavily traveled highways. Consultation with representatives of industry and highway departments may prove valuable.
4. Future plans with regard to the overall size of the hospital. Growth of activity in a department has a habit of paralleling overall hospital activity.

5. Other hospital construction in the area.

6. Trends in the makeup of the hospital staff. If it has been predominantly a staff of general practitioners, is there a swing toward a higher percentage of specialists, particularly surgical specialists?

7. Versatility of medical staffs in other hospitals within easy reach.

It is quite evident that before anyone sits down to a drawing board, the group as a whole must do some careful analyzing, some predicting, and even some soul-searching. Dreaming should be kept to a minimum. It would be easy for an enthusiastic but poorly informed trustee to be carried away by what he has seen in a superficial visit elsewhere. He might also be easily influenced by a doctor who pictured great strides in the quantity and quality of medical care simply because of the installation of much of the newest technical equipment. There are such doctors, and they have been known to wield much influence. Nothing is to be gained by spending thousands of dollars on the construction of facilities and purchase of equipment beyond the ability of the staff to use. A hospital is more likely to lay itself open to criticism and litigation by giving the impression that it is equipped for any eventuality when it is not, than it is if it provides only the equipment which its staff can use intelligently and within the bounds of safety. Any program of the hospital to increase the versatility of its staff by encouraging trained specialists is praiseworthy, but such a program should precede the acquisition of material things. These may be added later as technical skills of the staff increase. These warnings are issued with the hope that they may prevent waste of funds that might better be channeled into other uses.

PLANNING BOARDS

The problems attendant upon construction of a new emergency department in an old hospital or in a new structure will differ in that the first may require some tearing down before building begins. However, the facilities needed will be the same, and we will consider the construction with the understanding that space is available and that the best use is to be made of it.

Hospital construction in more and more areas of the United States is being influenced by area planning boards or councils. These may be city-wide, state-wide, or of intermediate size. While the planning boards have not yet had enthusiastic acceptance by all, particularly by all physicians, the principle is sound. Community pride is a virtue if curbed by realistic conservatism. Planning boards can aid in the development of the latter. Where they have been organized as a result of a need felt by the hospitals in the area, they are more likely to function effectively than if they have been developed through the efforts of other agencies and have attempted to dictate to hospital boards and communities. It is only natural that the large sources of financial support for hospital construction should desire objective opinion regarding the need for such construction. When the need for emergency department facilities capable of carrying the present and predictable future work loads has been confirmed, and the committee has determined the general policies, it is time for the drawing board.

The committee has then reached the stage where floor plans should be prepared, and the architect must not only be present but his advice must be seriously considered. Time will be saved, however, if someone looks over his shoulder as he sketches. Much is to be gained by having him meet with the committee long before this. He will welcome this opportunity. Anyone who has followed the building or remodeling of a hospital knows that mistakes are easily made. Some are quite obvious the minute the hospital is put to use; many of these could be avoided if more thought were given to function. Architects cannot be expected to know these things in advance. Administrators, but particularly doctors and nurses, do know them, and their advice must be blended with the architect's skill.

Suggestions have been presented with regard to the physical entrance to the department and the location of the nurse's station. A list of other desirable features that may be presented to the architect follows:

1. Reception area; lobby or corridor.
2. Examination and treatment area.
3. Operating room.
4. Fracture or cast room.
5. Eye, ear, nose, and throat room.
6. Cardiac room.
7. Poison center.
8. Visitor's waiting room.
9. Toilets and telephones.
10. Doctor's room.
11. Observation ward or rooms.
12. Security room.
13. Laboratory.
14. Diet kitchen or pantry.
15. Supply and utility rooms.
16. Morgue.
17. Room for police, press, and ambulance crews.
18. Space for wheelchairs and stretchers.

These facilities have not been listed in the order of importance but so that they will be considered. Not all are essential, and several may not be practical in some hospitals, but they will be discussed.

Reception Area

The entrance door will lead into a corridor or lobby. The shape and size of this must be determined in relation to the overall plan. While in some cases this may be used as a triage area, its main function is a passageway to the area where patients are examined and treated. It should be spacious enough to provide seats for ambulatory patients who may have to wait until more seriously injured stretcher patients have received attention, unless a waiting room is provided. A separate waiting room for patients and friends is much better.

In places such as the Louisville General Hospital, where all seriously injured patients requiring surgery are sent immediately to the operating room suite, this area may serve mainly as a passageway to the elevators. The unique situation in Louisville is discussed further in the section devoted to operating rooms.

Examination and Treatment Area

This, of course, is the center of most importance. It must be ready at all times for the reception of acutely ill or seriously injured patients. It is this area that must not be overrun by nonemergent patients if the department is to serve its real function. Suggestions are given elsewhere for plans to prevent this. It is assumed here that the planning committee is thinking in terms of the care of emergencies.

Many opinions have been expressed as to how this area should be laid out. Some who have expressed opinions have defended their stand with something short of full conviction. Granted that usable space, allotted funds, available personnel, and other factors will influence construction plans, it is difficult for anyone to offer valid arguments against a wide-open treatment area with stretchers separated only by curtains. Some who have not had the opportunity to work in shock wards or tents in military hospitals may be reluctant to accept this concept of a treatment area, but they too can see its advantages in most situations.

The extreme opposite to this type of construction is a series of private treatment rooms opening off one or both sides of a corridor. This looks beautiful to the uninitiated and, we might add, to the unwary. It offers the maximum of privacy to the individual patient. It would impress the members of a service club or a ladies auxiliary, particularly if the complete equipment in each room was pointed out. If this equipment could include a doctor and a nurse in each room, much of the objection to this type of construction would be invalidated, but not all. Such departments have been planned and constructed only to be condemned when put into use. In one large city hospital, this error was so serious that a completely new department was planned and constructed, and the private room setup was abandoned and turned over to the outpatient department.

The great majority of hospitals in this country do not have a staff of interns and residents. Neither do they have a full platoon of nurses available for the emergency department. It is evident that a doctor and a nurse will not be available for each occupied room. Many of these hospitals admit to their emergency departments a number of severely injured people at one time. Some of these may obviously be in critical condition, while others may have such injuries that their condition may become critical if they are not given prompt supportive therapy. It is of paramount importance that all of these patients be kept under constant observation. Priorities of treatment may have to be altered after the initial assessment. A limited nursing and medical staff cannot keep all the patients under observation, let alone promptly treat them, if they are relegated to rooms where they are out of sight and probably out of sound.

Much attention has been given to the multiple injury patient. Possibly not enough has been given to the multiple patient accident. When the two are combined, a situation is created calling for a mustering of all forces and a maximum conservation of all resources. The scattering of a number of critically injured patients through a series of isolated rooms defeats this purpose and reduces the effectiveness of the overall effort. Robben,[1] of Silver Springs, Maryland, has said, "While I am taking care of one injured patient, I want to listen to the breathing of that other patient and see how he is doing."

The answer to this is the open emergency ward where even one physician may make an overall estimate of the situation and have some idea as to where to start. Aided by several nurses, he will be able to carry out supportive measures and definitive treatments and still direct other activities. As he is joined by other members of the staff, if they are available, much time and duplication of effort may be saved by his brief report on each patient to his colleagues. Curtains may be temporarily drawn to provide any essential privacy during examinations, but the important feature is diagnosis and treatment, not social considerations. Few severely injured patients will object, but they will object to temporary abandonment behind walls.

In discussing the two types of construction, Shortliffe[2] states "Although solid partitions give maximum privacy they do destroy the full flexibility desired in the department." In presenting the argument for a wide, curtained space, he mentions the ability to convert it into a triage area. This is sound thinking, and he adds that the physical facilities should "be designed to conserve as much energy and time as possible."

This is particularly true in the majority of hospitals in this country lacking a resident staff, but even the availability of a full quota of residents did not make those in charge of the emergency department at the Montreal General Hospital happy with their new partitioned facility. They have given other reasons for the open area. Dickison[3] has told the story as follows:

> To meet today's requirements, firmly entrenched views on the planning of emergency services must change. *A large unobstructed space with all modern treatment facilities is necessary.** A radiological unit adjacent to such a department is as essential as oxygen and suction equipment. Rapid diagnosis and treatment are of paramount importance, and such a department must be equipped to deal with the acute medical emergency as well as the acute surgical patient.
>
> When the Montreal General Hospital moved to its present site in 1956, every effort was made to provide the best accommodation and latest equipment for the care of the sick. Each of the Hospital's services was given a major part in the development of plans for the areas of its interest. Layout of the emergency-casualty department was done with the guidance of the then chief surgeon, and this, as will be seen in accompanying plan, provided two operating theatres, seven examination rooms and a dressing room. (Fig. 10A)
>
> It soon became clear, however, that these facilities were inadequate to handle the increasing number of emergencies being brought in to the Montreal General. In addition to the normal difficulties in tending the sick, complaints were received over delayed treatment. People were waiting several hours for x-rays of minor injuries to joints; the severely injured patient was being treated in the constricted space of a small room, and ordinary minor emergency cases undergoing treatment frequently filled all available space, making it difficult to place the severely sick.
>
> In late 1959, under the direction of the surgeon-in-chief, Dr. H. Rocke Robertson, a study was undertaken to see how this situation

---

* Author's italics.

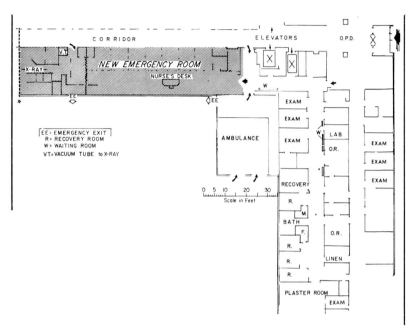

Figure 10A. Old emergency department floor plan at Montreal General Hospital. Divided into small rooms. The shaded area is new department.

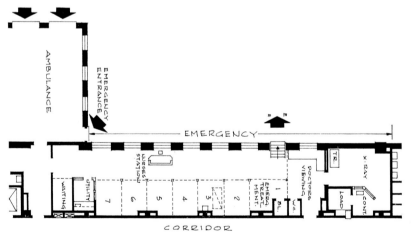

Figure 10B. New emergency department floor plan at Montreal General Hospital. The large treatment area where seven stretchers are separated by curtains is shown. Architects: McDougall, Smith, and Fleming (Montreal).

could be corrected. After visiting various other centers in Canada and the United States, the decision was made to take over another section of this floor as a new emergency room. The added space thus obtained is shown in the shaded area on the floor plan. (Fig. 10A and 10B)

This room (Fig. 11) ready for use in late 1961 is situated with direct access to the ambulance entrance. It has seven complete bed units with recovery room beds and all the necessary fixtures for resuscitative care. Each unit is equipped with vaporized oxygen, suction, examining lamp and wall sphygmomanometer. At the far end of this area a complete x-ray unit has been installed with a direct-line pneumatic tube for transferring x-rays to the automatic Xomat x-ray processing machine which is situated five floors above. As an average of 28 cases a day is handled in this room, 1500 to 2000 plates are processed here each month.

The advantage of having a single large well-illuminated, airy room for emergency care cannot be over-emphasized. *Draw curtains provide all the privacy that is required for this type of patient. There is plenty of working room for the treatment of a patient with multiple injuries where the need for adequate space is obvious.*[*] The entire area can be kept immaculate by the house-keeping staff as the floor can be cleaned from one end of the room to the other without any division of space.

In discussing the arrangement of the emergency department treatment area in Curry's book on transportation of the injured, Skudder[4] states, "Curtains are the least desirable, since they

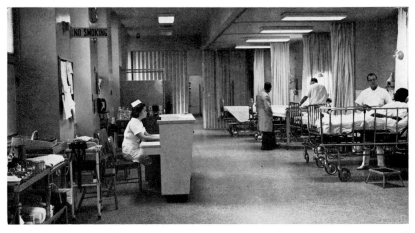

Figure 11. Curtained treatment area in emergency department, Montreal General Hospital, Montreal, Quebec.

* Author's italics.

are the least soundproof, they collect dust and they provide the least privacy."

Dickison,[5] however, says, ". . . our curtains, which are changed periodically and are always fresh, clean and neat can be moved right out of the way or can be used to make a double enclosed room or used singly for the seven separate units." Possibly the Canadians are better housekeepers!

In the next paragraph, Skudder points up the advantage of the open, curtained area when he says, "For emergency departments receiving many critically ill or injured patients requiring constant observation, the open or shock ward arrangement is most desirable, with a sorting area close to the entrance of the department." Surely any emergency department must expect to have such admissions from time to time. No one will take issue with the construction of a few individual examination and treatment rooms if the basic facility is the "open or shock ward arrangement."

Gurd,[6] who is now surgeon-in-chief at Montreal General Hospital, agrees with Dickison that patients do not complain of lack of privacy and that their new arrangement makes for maximum efficiency, for it not only allows observation of all patients but provides room for equipment that could not be used in private rooms.

It will be seen that a full quota of doctors and nurses still does not bring the efficiency of the private treatment rooms up to that of the open area. The very hospitals where funds, space, and staff might suggest the advisability of the private room system are the same places that will probably have available the equipment to which Gurd refers, as well as the skilled personnel to use it. Is it fair to deprive patients of the use of such equipment in the name of transient privacy? An interest in the patients' welfare suggests a negative answer.

The use of the curtained cubicles at the Chilton Memorial Hospital, Pompton Plains, New Jersey, is also shown in Figure 27. They report it as highly successful and much better than private rooms.*

* The Chilton Hospital has just opened a new emergency department in a new building. They have retained the curtained cubicles and now have nine.

Various compromises between the private rooms and the open area have been devised; one compromise is to have both. The John Gaston Memorial Hospital in Memphis, Tennessee, has one of the most comprehensive emergency departments this writer has seen. It not only has private treatment and examination rooms but has some of these equipped for special purposes, such as suturing and application of casts (see Fig. 12 for floor plan). When being shown through this department by Dr. Roger T. Sherman, the author was impressed with the definitive planning and the attention to details but was disappointed that he had not seen an area where a number of stretcher patients could be admitted and observed at the same time. He expressed his concern as tactfully as possible, only to have Dr. Sherman reply, "Wait, you haven't seen our hot spot yet." We had traversed one corridor known as the "yellow concourse" and had seen the rooms opening from it. We then started down the "grey concourse" and entered a large area, 23 × 45 feet, with a series of seven special emergency department stretchers separated only by draw curtains, hung on traverse rods in such a way as to allow any or all of the stretchers to be excluded from general view as desired (see Fig. 13). On the wall at the head of each stretcher was the required equipment, such as sphygmomanometers, suction, oxygen, and other equipment needed in the care of each patient, and at the foot of each stretcher was a stand on castors. Two-way intercom equipment was inserted in the wall at each stretcher area.

This area was easily accessible from the emergency department entrance and was for the reception of a number of patients at one time and the treatment of many of them. The small rooms were for special procedures and were to be used when sufficient staff was available. It is interesting to note that the original architect's plan of this open "hot spot" area had it divided up by several partitions which fortunately were vetoed before construction began.

Another compromise which provides semiprivacy without isolation is solid partitions between the stretchers, with curtains that may be drawn across the end of the booths thus

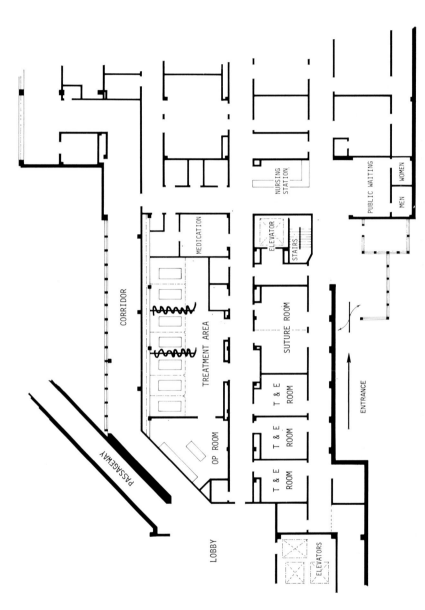

Figure 12. Floor plan of part of the emergency department, John Gaston Memorial Hospital, University of Tennessee, Memphis, Tennessee. This shows small treatment rooms and a large treatment area with seven stretchers. The wavy lines in the treatment area show where partitions in the original plan were removed by the committee. Architect: Walk C. Jones, Jr. (Memphis).

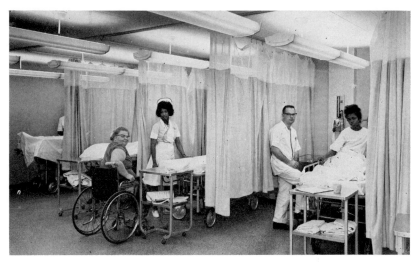

Figure 13. Curtained treatment area in emergency department, John Gaston Memorial Hospital, Memphis, Tennessee.

formed. Figure 14 shows the treatment area in the emergency department of the University of West Virginia Hospital, which has this type of construction. With the curtains drawn back, the patients in the several booths may be seen from a position across the room in front of the very well planned storage cabinets and working shelves. This department shows superior preconstruction planning, and the staff is pleased with it. Probably few teaching hospitals in this country were in the planning stage as long as that at Morgantown, West Virignia, and the benefits of careful planning are evident on all sides.

The partitions between stretchers need not be ceramic tile as shown here. They may be made of corrugated plastic material or even of frosted glass.

The open area has proved so completely satisfactory to those using it that it should always be considered in planning. A number of instances are known where the medical and nursing staffs have wished that the emergency department had not been completely partitioned, but dissatisfaction with the open area has yet to be reported. Montreal is not the only place where the private rooms have been abandoned.

The open area or shock-ward type of construction has found

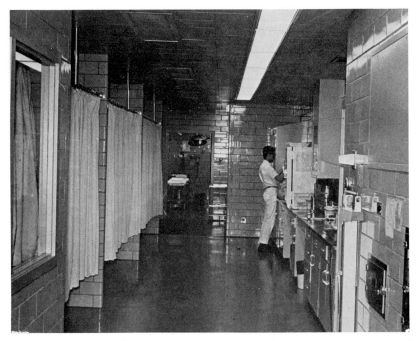

Figure 14. Curtained cubicles in emergency department, University of West Virginia Hospital, Morgantown, West Virginia. Supply cabinets, work shelf, sink, and x-ray viewing box are opposite the cubicles.

favor in countries other than the United States and Canada. The author has seen it in a number of hospitals in Europe. Figure 15 shows this type of construction in the Accident Hospital, founded by Lorenz Böhler, in Vienna, Austria. Dr. Emil Beck, who was a splendid guide through this institution, pointed out that there were really three rooms for the receipt of patients. One was for seriously injured patients on stretchers, one for walking injured, and a third for minor injuries needing suture. All were built to accommodate several patients, with curtains between the stretchers. No private treatment rooms were seen. At the Arbeitsunfalkrankenhaus, in Linz, Austria, also devoted to the care of accidents and where Jorg Böhler is chief, the pattern followed that of the parent institution in Vienna.

In England, the idea of an entire hospital being used for accidents has also been put into practice in several places. One

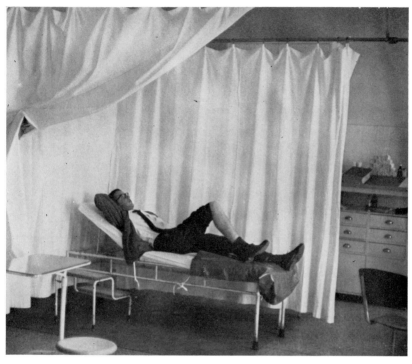

Figure 15. Curtained cubicles in treatment room, Vienna Accident Hospital, Austria.

of these, the Birmingham Accident Hospital, has two entrances for injured. The severely injured ambulance patients are taken directly into the Major Injuries admission room, where immediate treatment can be given. Figure 16 shows the interior of this room, with the patient's entrance at the right. Mr. D.M. Jackson, F.R.C.S.,[7] describes this room as having "all equipment which may be necessary for immediate resuscitation, passage of endotracheal tubes, emergency splintage, x-ray, anesthesia and artificial respiration." He states that the supply of first class nurses for care of patients admitted here comes from the adjacent Intensive Care Ward. This ward, with its curtain partitions, is shown clearly in Figure 17. Mr. Jackson says that it contains four beds, but they would like it to contain more. In describing the room further, he states that "these beds are usually filled with unconscious patients, multiple

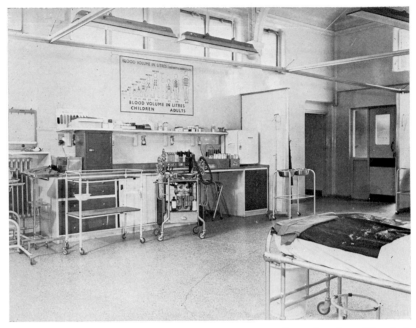

Figure 16. Major injuries admission room, Birmingham Accident Hospital, Birmingham, England.

injury patients and patients with severe chest and abdominal injuries. As soon as they are sufficiently recovered, they are transferred to one of the general wards. The staff from this Intensive Care Unit can be diverted next door to the Major Injuries admission room at a moment's notice when required. Male and female are mixed in both the wards with only a curtain between."

The other patients' entrance leads into what is termed the Casualty Department, for less severely ill or injured patients. This is described by Mr. Jackson as, ". . . again a row of cubicles made by curtaining a large room." Figure 18 shows this room from the entrance end. The door at the far end leads into a corridor through which patients may be taken to "short stay" wards, one each for males and females. Other facilities provided are an emergency operating theatre; x-ray department; plaster room; toilets; telephones; kitchen; room for re-dressings; waiting room for relatives; offices for surgeons, nursing sisters, and secretaries; record room; and even a photo-

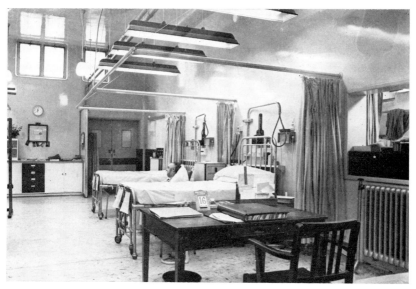

Figure 17. Intensive care ward, Birmingham Accident Hospital, Birmingham, England. This is adjacent to the major injuries admission room. The major injuries room is staffed from the intensive care ward when patients arrive.

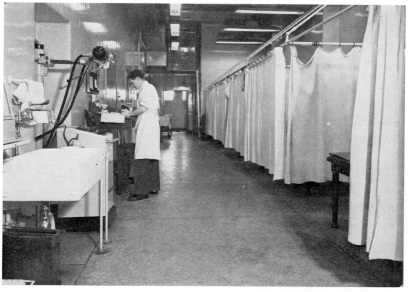

Figure 18. Curtained cubicles in the casualty department, Birmingham Accident Hospital, Birmingham, England. Less severe injuries are treated here, rather than in the major injuries room.

graphic department. Planning to make the maximum use of personnel is everywhere in evidence.

Justice would not be done the emergency facilities in Birmingham without reference to the ambulances which are operated by the city and parked in front of the Accident Hospital ready for instant use. The author was impressed with the fact that they did not give the impression of having been built for speed or beauty. They are functional. One of these is shown in Figure 19, and Figure 20 shows the interior. They are roomy, have high ceilings, and can carry several patients. The equipment is superior and easily accessible.

The Radcliffe Infirmary in Oxford, under the jurisdiction of the United Oxford Hospitals' Accident Service, has one of the best emergency departments in England. The entrance to this department was shown in Figures 4 and 5 in Chapter 2. In Figure 21, which is a floor plan of this department, the area numbered *20* is used for most emergency admissions. The curtained concept is shown in Figure 22. This large room will accommodate several patients at the same time. If privacy is required for certain examinations, the cubicles numbered *6* in the floor plan and shown in Figure 23 provide privacy. The surgical registrar who showed the author around in May, 1965,

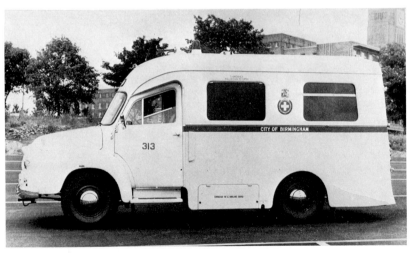

Figure 19. City of Birmingham (England) ambulance.

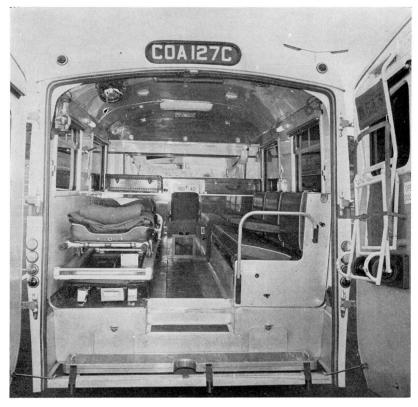

Figure 20. City of Birmingham ambulance (interior).

explained that severely injured patients requiring resuscitation were taken through a separate entrance into Room 13 on the floor plan. Here the department of anesthesiology has complete equipment for treating shock as well as for administering anesthesia. It was pointed out that if there were several such critical patients, they might overflow into the adjoining plaster room (Fig. 24) and still have close at hand all of the facilities for resuscitation. The planning of the department demonstrated thought as to flexibility and maximum function under varying conditions.

It seems clear that those who have had wide experience in the use of facilities caring for a heavy load of emergency patients, particularly those with injuries, find the open-area or

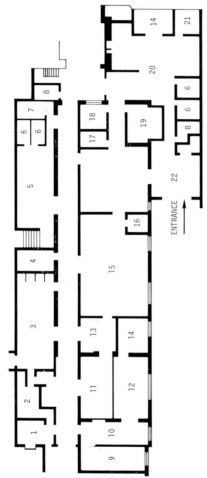

Figure 21. Floor plan of casualty department, Radcliffe Infirmary, Oxford, England. Rooms referred to in the text are (6) examination cubicles, (13) anesthetic room, (15) plaster room, and (20) curtained treatment area. Architects: J.F. Watkins and Partners (Oxford).

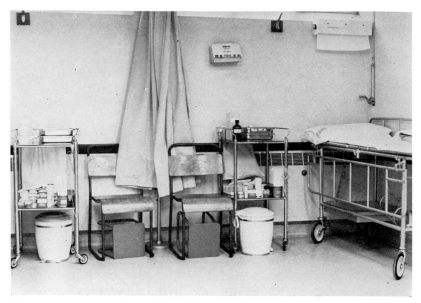

Figure 22. Curtained treatment area, casualty department, Radcliffe Infirmary, Oxford, England.

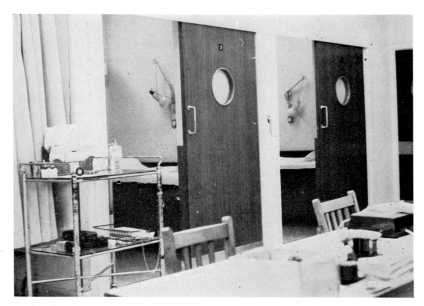

Figure 23. Closed cubicles, casualty department, Radcliffe Infirmary, Oxford, England.

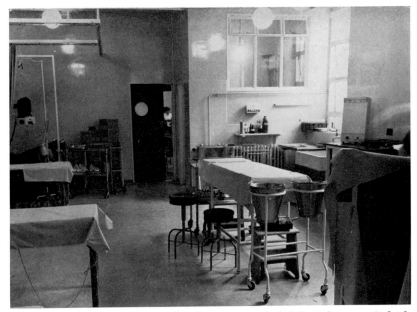

Figure 24. Plaster room, casualty department, Radcliffe Infirmary, Oxford, England.

shock-ward concept of construction most satisfactory. No objection can be advanced to the construction of several individual treatment rooms where space is available, but they should not replace the more functional section of the department. To suggest that the whole department should be so divided because most of the admissions are "private" patients is to do an injustice to such patients. They are deserving of just as good care as the indigent. The slogan *Preservation before Privacy* might well be adopted in the planning.

Whichever plan is followed, built-in features on the wall at the head of each stretcher are an asset (see Fig. 25). In new construction, it is not difficult to install suction and piped oxygen in the walls, as well as electric outlets. Wall sphygmomanometers, with tubing of adequate length, are an improvement over the portable or even the stand type. At Montreal General (Fig. 26), running water is provided at the head of each stretcher, although conveniently located sinks may be so placed as to serve several stretchers in large areas.

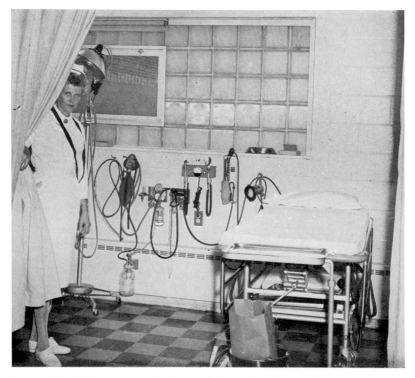

Figure 25. Chilton Memorial Hospital, Pompton Plains, New Jersey, emergency department. Emergency utilities are shown on the wall next to each stretcher.

When private rooms are built either alone or to supplement the large area, they should all have oxygen, suction, and running water. The same is true of cabinet space for at least a minimum of supplies in each room. A nurse does not have time to leave the room when attending a critical patient. The most efficient types of cabinet and work-shelf arrangements are those shown in the photograph of Chilton Memorial Hospital, Pompton Plains, New Jersey (Fig. 27). This also illustrates the curtained treatment area. Figure 28 shows the same type of cabinet arrangement at the University of West Virginia Hospital. The supplies in the cabinets in both of these departments are a minimum of steps away from any of the stretchers in the room.

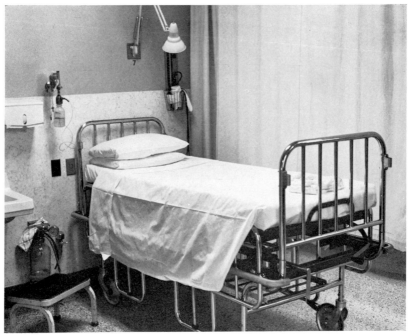

Figure 26. Montreal General Hospital, Montreal, Quebec, emergency department. Running water as well as other utilities are located next to each of the seven stretchers.

Operating Room

Some maintain that an emergency department should have no operating room. It is their contention that any patient needing surgery beyond simple suturing or the reduction of a closed fracture should be moved to the operating room suite in the hospital. They support this stand with sound arguments, such as the difficulty of maintaining sterility in an O.R. in this area, the necessity of keeping a room equipped and supplied when it may not be used regularly, the problem of providing adequate anesthesia service, as well as other things. No doubt, those who hold this view are in the right with respect to their particular institutions.

Noer[8] feels that any patient requiring anything but the simplest surgical procedure, and even those requiring transfusion, should go immediately to the operating suite. Horan[9]

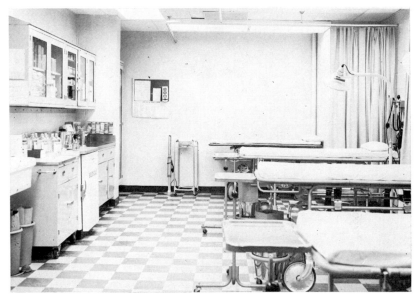

Figure 27. Chilton Memorial Hospital, Pompton Plains, New Jersey, emergency department. Convenient supply cabinets, work shelves, and sink are located opposite the stretchers, which are separated by curtains.

describes the procedure in the Louisville General Hospital where Noer works. In her visit there, she saw the emergency room doctor examine patients at the entrance and send the severely injured ones directly to a special room in the operating room suite. Looking at this from a nurse's viewpoint, she observes that this "frees the emergency room nurses for care of less critically ill patients." Noer[10] admits, however, that the operating suite in his hospital is staffed around the clock and that their plan might not be the best under some circumstances. The author has visited Louisville General Hospital and is convinced that the superior ambulance service of the police in that city, plus the system of handling injured patients at the hospital, offers the citizens of that community a maximum opportunity to recover from critical injuries.

There are hospitals where the administration of the nursing service, the wishes of the attending staff, and the availability of anesthesia service make an operating room an asset in the

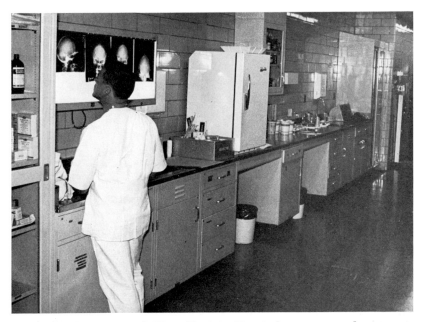

Figure 28. University of West Virginia Hospital emergency department. Built-in supply cabinets, refrigerator, sink, and x-ray view boxes are located opposite the stretchers, which are in curtained cubicles.

emergency department suite. The planning committee will need to weigh all of the evidence to arrive at a sound decision. One thing that should be insisted upon is that the same rigid standards apply here as in the regular operating rooms. Surgery in an emergency department should not be considered as secondary in importance, and the patients should have the protection of rigid controls equal to those applied elsewhere in the hospital. Size should not be compromised. The same rules of safety should apply. If there is any possibility that explosive anesthetic agents will be used, the floor should be conductive. Adequate lighting should be provided. Supply cabinets planned to store supplies for this room only should be installed. These supplies should not be interchangeable with those in other parts of the department. The floor, and particularly the baseboards, should be free from cracks and dirt-catching recesses and should be easily cleaned. There should be scrub sinks apart from those in the rest of the department. In short, the room should satisfy the critical conscientious surgeon who may have to operate there.

Fracture or Cast Room

This is a room equipped for closed reduction of fractures and application of casts. An occasional opinion against this room is also expressed. The voluminous correspondence preceding the publication of the emergency department brochure by the American Hospital Association shows one big-city orthopedist objecting to a fracture room. This is another example of a viewpoint based on narrow experience. He works in a large county hospital where there are no doubt "hungry" orthopedic residents eager to whisk fracture patients off to a completely equipped orthopedic department at any time of the day or night. This situation is not typical of most hospitals in the United States and Canada. If space is available, a fracture room is truly an asset. If it can be constructed so as to open directly into the large treatment area, as it does at the Chilton Memorial Hospital (Fig. 29), it will serve as an expan-

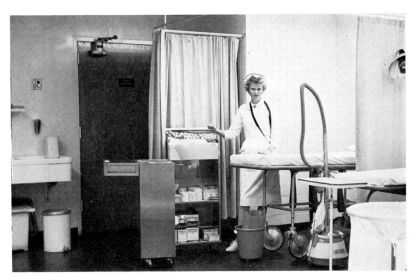

Figure 29. Chilton Memorial Hospital, Pompton Plains, New Jersey, fracture room. While equipped for plaster application, this room opens into the main treatment room and may be used for any type of patient.

sion to that area when needed for other than fracture patients. This also fulfills Shortliffe's[2] criteria, when he pleads that "specific areas for plaster application or the management of acute nose and eye emergencies should be available for treatment of other types of cases."

Any open reductions will be done in the operating room suite or in the emergency department operating room. Size should not be skimped in the cast room either. There must be room for a fracture table or at least a table that is solid and has attachments to support extremities during reductions. There must also be room for several straight chairs and a portable x-ray machine, although built-in x-ray equipment is better. Here again, if it is planned to use explosive gases in anesthesia, the floor should be conductive. Ceiling pulleys, strategically located with relation to the fracture table, are an asset. Unless the fracture table has a suspension arm that will hold the weight of a patient during the application of a body cast, at least one of the ceiling pulleys should be rugged enough to serve this purpose.

Closets or cabinets to house a variety of splints, plaster bandages, and other fracture accessories will complete the features to be considered in construction. Good illumination must be provided, although an operating room light is not needed.

Although the writer agrees in principle with the statement in the American Hospital Association brochure that the emergency department should not be used for the treatment of inpatients, the changing of casts might be an exception to this. Small hospitals may find it wasteful to have duplicate facilities of this type. If there is a room designated for an orthopedic clinic, this is a better place for scheduled changing of casts. This keeps the nonemergencies out of the emergency department.

Eye, Ear, Nose, and Throat Room

This room is mentioned largely because of tradition. There is actually little reason to provide a separate room for patients in these categories unless the department is doubling as an outpatient department. It does not require a hydraulic chair to look into little Sally's throat, particularly if it is only to determine if she should have her tonsils out come Spring. Instruments for the diagnosis and treatment of conditions in these specialties should, of course, be available, but a separate room seems hardly necessary. Capability of darkening one of the other rooms will be advisable.

Cardiac Room

See Chapter 16 for complete discussion.

Poison Center

One of the most serious of medical emergencies is the swallowing of poisons. A card index of poisons with the appropriate antidotes will be most valuable. In spite of controlling laws, it is inevitable that certain poisons be used in the average household. Adults will usually avoid ingesting these, but children may not. Such household poisons as well as those used in factories or other community installations should be included in the index. A book on toxicology, as mentioned in the chapter on equipment, should be available. There are organized poison centers in most areas in this country offering around-the-clock telephone information on the treatment of poisons. Unusual poisons, not included in the index, are known to these centers, and the telephone number of the nearest information center should be posted in a prominent place in such a way that it will not be mislaid or covered up.

Visitors' Waiting Room

This feature is practically essential to prevent unauthorized people from crowding into the treatment area. The handling of these people is discussed in the chapter entitled "People and Problems." Visitors cannot be expected to stay out of the treatment area unless there is a place to wait. This room should not have unobstructed vision into the treatment area. Well-meaning, but troublesome, family and friends should not be tempted to interfere with treatment. The waiting room should be comfortably furnished, and a supply of reading material will prove worthwhile.

Toilets and Telephones

These should be readily available and clearly marked. A pay-station booth is the best location for the telephone; an open pay telephone is not so satisfactory. Police and press as well as friends and family will appreciate privacy.

Doctors' Room

If the hospital has a resident staff, and particularly if the department is so busy that residents or interns are assigned there full-time for certain hours, they need a room in which to read, relax, and—if on night shift—sleep. If there are no residents, but members of the attending staff stay in the hospital at night as required by law in some states, they need a room. This should have toilet facilities, be well ventilated, and be provided with a bed, a desk, and at least two comfortable chairs. At times, doctors, may use this room when they confer with consultants or talk to patients, family, or friends.

Observation Ward or Rooms

It may be difficult to decide, after some patients are treated in the emergency department, whether they may be safely sent home or not. Admission to the hospital may not seem necessary, but the attendant may wish to defer his decision on this. Patients with mild cerebral concussion, abdominal contusion, or acute alcoholism may fall into this classification. A place to detain them for a few hours or overnight may avoid the trouble and expense of formal admission to the hospital and yet protect them against delayed deteriorization with its dangers. A detention ward with curtains between beds will fill the need for patients of both sexes for short stays, or two single or double rooms may be provided. This facility may also serve as a recovery ward after short anesthesias. The University of Mississippi Hospital has seen fit to provide many more of these beds than treatment units. There are twelve in the emergency department at the Johns Hopkins Hospital. The limit for occupancy in the latter institution is 48 hours. Both of these hospitals have many emergency patients whose final disposition may not be easy to determine immediately. The nature of the patient population and the hospital admission policy will influence the planning of holding or observation beds.

Some who argue against an observation room or area do not fully understand its function. It is not an intensive care unit per se, where constant nursing attention would be required. If a patient calls for this, he should, of course, be admitted. An observation room can be adjoining the general treatment area with the doorway or passageway open, and a nurse or doctor should go in periodically and check the progress of the patient or patients. Improvement or lack of it may be noted, so that later a decision may be made as to whether the patient should be admitted. Periodic observation by the same doctor who saw the patient originally is more meaningful than that of someone else without first-hand knowledge of the earlier condition. This need not take much time, and bedside records of vital signs and other information can be kept without neglect of care of new patients coming in. Of course, if the nursing staff is large enough and there are several patients in the room, it may be advisable to assign a nurse there regularly. The exact amount of personnel needed in an active emergency department can never be determined ahead of time. It will vary with each day and hour.

Security Room

Some patients, acutely intoxicated or in an otherwise unmanageable state, may not be fit candidates for the observation ward or rooms. The interests of other patients should be considered, and they should not be subjected to the indignities of association with these unfortunate individuals who at least temporarily are not acceptable members of society. Such patients may well be put in a room having no table or chairs and either a low bed or only a mattress. It must be remembered that the prospective inmates of this room are irresponsible, and all precautions should be taken to prevent them from injuring themselves or others. The door of this room should lock from the outside but not from the inside, and a small plate-glass window may be provided in the door for attendants to view the condition of the patient. The walls and ceiling should be sound absorbing. Worthylake and Branch discuss the use of this room in the chapter, "Psychiatric Patient in the Emergency Room." They outline some practical precautions to be taken.

Laboratory

Unless the hospital clinical laboratory is staffed around the clock, a small laboratory for simple blood and urine examinations will save unnecessary demands on the laboratory staff. This need only be a shelf in a corner where urine may be tested for sugar and albumin and where hemoglobin determinations may be done. Any extensive laboratory tests should be done by the regular laboratory technicians in the main laboratory. A very large and active emergency department may justify the planning of a more versatile and permanently staffed laboratory.

Diet Kitchen or Pantry

Here again, the provision of such a facility will depend on the service available at night from the regular hospital kitchen. If the kitchen is closed, provision for at least coffee and toast is a great asset. It will be appreciated by staff putting in long hours unexpectedly and will enhance the public relations of the hospital. Anxious friends and relatives as well as ambulance attendants and police will not forget any gestures to make them more comfortable. Coin-operated coffee or snack vending machines will be convenient additions.

Supply and Utility Rooms

While a supply room is no substitute for well-stocked cabinets within easy reach of the patients' stretchers, if the department is a large one, it may be decided to store reserve supplies in a separate room. From this room, the working cabinets may be restocked. The nursing service or other designated authority from central supply will keep this room stocked. There should be a running inventory here and in the supply cabinets.

The supply room may also serve as a utility room unless the department is large enough to justify a separate one. Provision may be made here for storage of patients' belongings under lock and key. With regard to locks, there is a difference of opinion as to what should be kept locked and what not. There are no arguments against keeping narcotics locked wherever they are stored, and in some places the law requires that they be double locked. The locking of cabinets in the supply room would seem to be a reasonable precaution. The locking of all cabinets in the working areas has the disadvantage of rendering certain supplies nonusable in an emergency, unless the keys are hanging alongside the cabinets. The locking of these cabinets with the keys in the possession of a nurse or other personnel is not logical, as this may result in the keys being out of the department when badly needed. This is a point that has resulted in friction between staff and administration and should be settled in such a way as to assure that there is no interference with patient care.

Morgue

The hospital morgue will usually suffice for patients coming in dead on arrival. It cannot be too strongly emphasized that where death is quite evident, bodies should not be brought into the emergency department. Arrangements should be made to take them to mortuaries or for other disposition. This should definitely be included in the hospital disaster plan.

Room for Police, Press, and Ambulance Crews

This will only be provided in larger departments, but is greatly appreciated when it is. It facilitates the control of the representatives of the press. It should never be forgotten that relationships with reporters are important in public relations of the hospital. This is discussed in some detail in the chapter on public relations. Both the reporters and the police will appreciate facilities set aside for them where the space justifies it, as will ambulance crews waiting for equipment.

Space for Wheelchairs and Stretchers

Patients who cannot walk but who do not need a stretcher may be brought to the hospital in private cars. Wheelchairs should be available for them. In addition to the stretchers permanently located in the treatment area, one or two should be stored near the entrance for the use of stretcher patients brought in trucks or other vehicles. If these stretchers are the same type as those in the treatment area, the patient will not be subjected to an extra shift from one stretcher to another. A room, an alcove, or simply an area in the lobby should be provided for these wheel chairs and stretchers so that they will be out of the way of traffic, yet always available (see Fig. 6).

SUMMARY

No suggestion is intended that all of these facilities are essential to a good emergency department. They are all useful when appropriate. The writer has seen them all in use, but seldom in the same place. Local needs will determine how elaborate the department should be from the standpoint of physical facilities.

The area of actual patient treatment is of course the most important of all, but this also must be planned on the basis of local circumstances. If after considering all factors the committee feels that the department should plan for an increasing number of nonemergency patients at any hour, the facilities should differ from those in a department planned specifically for emergency care. The operation of what is essentially a complete outpatient service under the guise of an emergency department will call for more partitioning and a different over-all plan. It is to be hoped that if such a service is considered, space will be available to provide it without using the one essential feature for emergency care, the "shock ward." This chapter on planning should be studied along with Chapter 1 on function, for a basic philosophy is woven into both.

REFERENCES

1. Robben, J.O.: Personal communication.
2. Shortliffe, E.C.: Emergency department. Some considerations on essential physical facilities. *Hospitals,* 36:48–125 *passim,* 1962.
3. Dickison, J.C.: New emergency room at the Montreal General Hospital. *Canadian Hospital,* Feb. 1963.

4. Skudder, P.A., and Wade, P.A.: The hospital emergency facility. In Curry, G.J.: *Immediate Care and Transportation of the Injured.* Springfield, Thomas, 1965.
5. Dickison, J.C.: Personal communication.
6. Gurd, F.N.: Personal communication.
7. Jackson, D.M.: Personal communication.
8. Noer, R.J.: Critical surgery belongs in O.R. not E.R. *Mod Hosp, 106:* 92–92, 1966.
9. Horan, P.D.: *RN, 1:*47–57, 1962.
10. Noer, R.J.: Personal communication.

Chapter 4

CONSTRUCTION

CHESTER H. PHILIPS

The term *construction,* as applied to the building of a new emergency department for a modern hospital, would appear to involve only the process—complex in itself to be sure—of converting the committee's stated needs into a finished product, by the routine of erecting steel or pouring concrete, applying roof, building walls, installing windows and partitions, and incorporating the necessary mechanical and electrical services and equipment needed for heat, light, and plumbing. However, like the proverbial iceberg which has two-thirds of its mass below the surface, the procedure that must be undertaken, the decisions made and approved, the technical details that must be analysed, the problems that must be solved, and the myriad of technical instructions that must be prepared first to make the construction process possible almost dwarf the physical, tangible, "bricks and mortar" phase.

This "unseen" part of the construction process, when detailed analysis and decisions must be made to implement the planning that has gone before, will inevitably make the difference between the highly efficient, successful result and one which never quite makes the grade. It is also the period when the greatest amount of cerebral activity on the part of all members of the planning team is necessary to ensure success. This thinking must be creative foresight, the most difficult kind, and not the critical type which finds it so easy to say, "It should not have been done this way; too bad we can't change it now." Because of the inordinate importance of this process in producing good results, most of this chapter will deal with it rather than the mixing of concrete or laying of bricks.

In this context, *construction* is essentially a continuation and extension of *Plans and Planning*, even up to the pouring of concrete and beyond, since more than a few times concepts have changed, mistakes been corrected, or better ideas been born *after* the bulldozers have started work, particularly in this age when critics can often state with considerable truth that a new hospital is obsolete before it opens its doors. Since this treatment, however, is surgery, it is to be hoped that the preventive medicine of intelligent analysis, careful planning, and good decisions will obviate its necessity.

In any case, when the building committee, with the full participation of its consultant (if one is a member of the planning team), its architect, and the emergency department staff, has gone through the thinking and planning process outlined in the previous chapter, the fruit of its labor will be a document which will state as requirements those portions of the various elements of emergency suites listed in Chapter 2 which are decided to be applicable to the specific needs of the specific hospital. This document will be labelled by the consultant and architect as the *Architectural Program* and will be the latter's bible during the design phase—his first major activity for the project, when he translates the requirements into a small-scale plan designed to show the committee in a general way how the final product will turn out. This so-called "schematic" plan,* the result of much effort and many trials, will give very basic information, such as the general layout of rooms and spaces; interrelations of functions; doors, walls, partitions; and a rough idea of major items of equipment, but probably will not show door swings, columns, mechanical or electrical equipment, nor many other vital aspects of a finished building. Since it will probably be part of a larger plan for the hospital, it will readily reveal, however, those very important aspects of general planning, such as relation to the other service areas, access and interior circulation, entrance approaches, and probably will be accompanied by some idea of exterior configuration. It may well have an inherent *implication* of a superior solution to the

---

* See Figure 30, *schematic drawing of an emergency department for a 500 bed hospital (1971).*

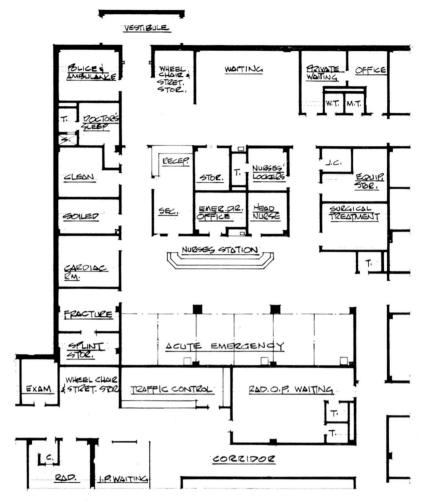

Figure 30. Schematic drawing of an emergency department for a 500-bed hospital (1971). Under construction at Morristown Memorial Hospital, Morristown, New Jersey. Architects: Epple and Seaman.

problem and could very well lead to the superficial thought that the matter can now be put aside and turned over to the architect for immediate conversion into a three dimensional reality. In this most complex of activities, alas, nothing could be more erroneous.

The approval of the schematic plan is by no means an assurance that the committee will get what it hopes to in the new facility. There are two other extremely important and time-consuming phases of the preliminary process to undergo before the building contractors can begin the "bricks and mortar" activities. The first of these is what the architect will call the design-development or preliminary phase. During this period he will re-draw the plans at a larger scale, usually at ⅛″ to the foot, and will "develop" in much greater detail the idea conveyed by the schematic drawing. Columns will appear (often where they are not wanted), and things like electrical closets and duct shafts will become a part of the plan, indicating that electrical and mechanical engineers are becoming part of the team. Door swings will be apparent and will often indicate problems not visualized before, and it is inevitable that numerous spaces which looked fine on the schematic now are undeniably too large or too small, too narrow or too wide. Such previously undiscussed items as ceiling height (for treatment room or surgical lights), type of ventilation, plumbing requirements (general anesthesia or not), casework (what cabinets in treatment rooms), and a host of others are now arising with remarkable multiplicity. The drawings will now show the arrangement of built-in and movable equipment in enough detail to convey just how the function of each space can be performed. At the time of the submission of the developed drawings, an outline specification will usually have been written, perhaps a more detailed edition of a very basic one presented with the schematic. This will present the type of structural system, walls, roof, floors, windows, partitions, doors, finishes, casework, equipment, electrical and mechanical systems that are proposed. Even highly condensed as it is in comparison with the later contract specifications, it can be a document difficult to absorb for many laymen, and a confusing anathema to a few. However, its importance cannot be overemphasized. When it is approved, a decision will have been made that may well affect the future of the department and the hospital. For example, if plastered masonry block partitions are specified throughout, changing the plan layout for future expansion may be next to impossible without putting the department out of business, whereas, in an area where flexibility is essential, metal partitions that snap in place and can be removed in a matter of hours are available at little or no greater cost and at no disadvantage in maintenance or aesthetics, acoustics or fire resistance; and steel-stud and plaster partitions have almost that ease of removability, are more economical, and have similar advantages, in addition to providing a better surface for certain finishes. In any event, approval of the outline specification should not be given until it has been thoroughly reviewed, explained, and understood. Once it has been approved, however, it will form the basis for contract documents, and when the latter are well under way, changes in basic decisions will be a serious cause of delay in completing the contract documents and could be a basis for extra compensation to the architect as a result if he is subjected thereby to do considerable corrective or extra work.

In evaluating the bewildering array of proposals submitted by the architect during the developed drawing* phase, the committee or those individuals charged by the hospital with responsibility for making the final decisions should keep several basic goals in mind, including the following:

1. *Long-term durability and ease of maintenance.* These qualities rarely come in the lowest price bracket of the available choices, but it can usually be demonstrated that the higher capital outlay can be amortized in a few years by savings in upkeep and replacement and reduced labor costs, not to mention the usual benefit of improved standards of patient care and safety. Of course, with the skyrocketing costs of hospital construction, all of these factors may be outweighed by first-cost considerations. Hospitals are prominent, tragically, among the many institutions and individuals with a "champagne taste and a beer pocketbook."

2. *Economy consistent with quality.* The constantly changing and developing aspects of the building materials field makes it extremely difficult for busy hospital people to keep up with the latest finishes available. But the importance of

* See Figure 31, an example of the "developed" plan of the emergency department of a 500-bed hospital.

such knowledge, which the competent hospital architect will have, is that often a time-honored and traditional material will have a competitor which is not only an improvement upon it, but is considerably less costly. A case in point is ceramic tile for use in operating rooms, until recently the standard finish. Today it is possible to obtain a vitreous finish equal to that of ceramic tile but without the joints that have always been a problem to keep clean, and at considerably less cost. Some of the new paints are a great improvement over the traditional types, and at lower cost. There are many other examples. It is advisable, however, to use caution in adopting new materials without evidence that they really represent quality. Most experienced architects will prefer that a new product have been installed successfully in demonstrable cases to avoid permitting a client to be the "guinea pig" whereby the unforeseen problems are worked out.

3. *Practical adaptability to the patient care function.* This should be perhaps listed first as being the most important. In essence, it is the most obvious, but is remarkably easy to overlook. Fundamentally, it involves the military commander's constant reminder to remember the nature of his mission and any problem-solver's time-honored reminder to go back and read the problem. It would be a sad waste of the hospital's limited funds to install a costly conductive floor in an emergency department without exploring to the limit its ability to perform its function without using flammable anesthetic agents.

4. *Flexibility.* The emergency department is one of the "explosive" ancillary departments of a modern hospital. Fitzimmons,[1] in a recent publication of the Public Health Service, has pointed out that the use of emergency facilities has increased on the average more than 112 percent in a decade. For this reason—and the obvious implications of burgeoning high-speed transportation; increasingly complex machinery in home and industry; ever-widening psychiatric, drug abuse, and other trauma-encouraging aspects of modern life—emergency departments should plan on the need for expansion, probably sooner than anyone can foresee. The planning should make it possible to add spaces and facilities, and if necessary to alter

existing ones, with the least possible interference with the concurrent functioning of the department. But this feature must be remembered through the developed drawing phase, for it is then that the details of easily removable exterior walls and designation of those interior partitions which can be made easily changeable are worked out. The use of "curtain wall" panels, prefabricated and bolted into place where corridors must extend in the future, will immeasurably assist in the ease with which such expansion will be accomplished. Adequate heating and ventilating capacity in pipes and ducts with provision for their extension; electric feeders available to extend to new panels without serious interruption of existing service; capped plumbing lines for water, medical gas, oxygen, suction, and other facilities should all be considered *now* in relation to the master plan for future expansion.

Not the least of the problems involved in planning for the future of the department will concern how to make possible adaptation to trends and changes in techniques and technology. This chapter will leave to the medical reader such of the latter as have to do with surgical and medical procedures affecting the department, but to overlook such foreseeable possibilities as helicopter transportation of highway accident and industrial accident trauma cases to emergency would be to deny a reality already in existence and attracting more attention every year. Increased use of diagnostic computer capabilities and electronic monitoring of an increasing number of parameters are less immediate but likely possibilities that could also have an effect upon planning for expansion, while the probability of highly sophisticated closed-circuit television capable of close supervision of patients' condition from a central location is likely enough within a few years to warrant consideration of the inclusion of empty conduits for the future wiring.

Not to be overlooked in the search for flexibility for future adaptation is the need for adequate space for utility lines, including those which may be needed later but not now. If the space between ceiling and roof construction is ample enough to permit the passage of ducts, pipes, and conduits, not only for the present construction but those which may be required in the future due to ever-increasing demands upon electrical power, or the need for more sophisticated communications, or more exotic medical gases, or refinements to heating, cooling, and ventilating requirements, the hospital owes a vote of thanks to the building committee, the architect, and all others responsible. The ceiling itself should be the easily removable type, permitting access to the utility space without difficulty. One of the most difficult hospital expansion problems encountered by the author involved a hospital built some fifteen years ago and widely publicized as a paragon of economical design and construction. Part of the savings in this low-cost construction, it was proclaimed, was due to the "sensible" design of minimal floor-to-floor heights (generally only ten feet), with acoustic ceilings attached by adhesive to the underside of the floor slab above. This "no wasted space" approach, while saving a few dollars initially, made it next to impossible fifteen years later to introduce efficient and modern air-conditioning systems into the structure, or to make any significant changes in the plumbing, or to make changes to conform with revised hospital building-code requirements in ventilation, or to pass large new electrical conduits through the existing structure to a new addition, or almost anything else except at great trouble and consequent exorbitant cost. The lesson, of course, is that the temptation to be penny wise and pound foolish in hospital construction must be countered by intelligent foresight.

Sooner or later during the developed drawing phase of the project, some sparkling idea on the part of a committee member or staff adviser, or possibly the consultant, will encounter a frustrating road block: the architect will announce that the building codes will not permit it. For hospital construction, compliance with municipal, state, and federal building requirements can be a complex and difficult problem. For the very sound reason that there have been some tragic catastrophes in hospitals as a result of fire, explosion, or accident, there has been a proliferation of building requirements aimed at producing foolproof safety conditions for patient care and the employees who perform it. And like most cases of unbridled exercise of police power, it occasionally is overdone, with the result that there are sometimes requirements that don't make much common sense and therefore do nothing to increase patient and staff safety. There is no question, however, that they contribute heavily to the high cost of hospital construction. To illustrate what the architect may be up against in the way of building code restrictions, in the *General Standards of Construction and Equipment for Hospital and Medical Facilities* publication of the U.S. Department of Health, Education, and Welfare, Public Health Service, which is itself very much a building code and is always in force for hospitals that have received a federal (Hill-Burton) construction grant, there is an interesting section entitled *Codes and Standards.* After a preliminary statement that nothing contained in the chapter "shall relieve the sponsor from compliance with building codes, ordinances and regulations which are enforced by city, county or State jurisdiction," it then proceeds to list no less than twenty codes and standards which have been "utilized in whole or in part as references in the sections of this publication. . . ."

But the end is not yet. In the state of New Jersey, as an example, there is a *New Jersey Supplementary Standards to the U.S. Public Health Service "General Standards"*, listing additional requirements imposed by the state, as well as state Department of Health regulations over water supply and sewage. Finally, there is the local municipality's building code, usually one of the standard codes such as the Building Code of the National Board of Fire Underwriters or the B.O.C.A. (Building Officials & Code Administrators) Code, which vary in their requirements considerably but are always quite specific about almost everything in a hospital, from the size and construction of stair enclosures and the direction in which doors must swing to the ventilation of storage rooms for medical gas containers. The answer to the obvious question as to which code will govern when there is a conflict is simple. *It is the most restrictive.* Superimposed upon all codes is the icing on the cake: the individual interpretations of them and the often purely whimsical personal requirements of the enforcing officials, the local building inspectors, and town engineers.

In many states, the Public Health Service requirements have been adopted as state requirements, so the multiple code complexity is present whether a federal grant is involved or not.

The outline specification will list a type of foundation and structural framework (usually concrete), type of roof, exterior walls, windows, if any, partitions, ceilings, floors, doors, casework, finishes in various areas, and special built-in hospital equipment (such as medicine preparation unit and sterilizer). The mechanical section of it will enumerate plumbing fixtures and describe systems for medical gases (if any), oxygen, suction, compressed air, type of heating and ventilating and air-conditioning systems. The electrical section will cover types of general and specialized lighting, types and locations of receptacles and outlets for special equipment such as portable radiological machines.

Decisions on these details will ultimately spell the difference between a successful unit and one that is inadequate to perform its function—one that is easy or difficult to maintain. It is therefore important to consider them in some detail with a few of the alternatives available.

Structural Frame

Due to highly restrictive fire protection regulations, the basic structural frame will generally be concrete. But, since concrete construction generally requires larger columns and narrower spans than steel construction, it is important that the structural engineer has designed a system that will reduce the number of columns to a minimum and will keep the spans as wide as the limitations of concrete design will permit. The roof system (or floor system, if floors are above) must also be designed to occupy as shallow a depth as possible so that maximum space may be left for the unencumbered passage of mechanical and electrical utility lines above the ceiling. Of course, there will be fewer columns and less problems imposed by the structural system if the department is housed in a one-story structure with no superimposed floors above. This, while it is an ideal situation not always attainable, is something to keep in mind when the schematics are presented. The usual structural solution is a "flat slab" (no beams are required) or a coffered or "waffle" slab supported by columns 20 to 25 feet apart. Depth of the horizontal components can be limited to as little as 14 inches.

Roof

Good insulation and a high-quality roofing are not to be compromised in the interests of economy. If the department is housed in a one-story wing, this is particularly important. Since the roof will normally be flat, the roofing is usually a bonded "composition" roof, made up of layers of impregnated "felts" mopped with pitch or asphalt and finished with slag or stone chips. A minimum of two inches of rigid insulation is placed under it, immediately upon the concrete slab. Adequate insulation is extremely important for comfort.

Exterior Walls

With a concrete frame, the exterior walls are non-loadbearing, and considerable flexibility is possible, with many alternatives. The time-honored dependable one is a masonry wall (built in two thicknesses, with mortar between or with a wide cavity between the "withes"), but while such a wall when properly built will often represent 100 years of weatherproof reliability, there are other dependable types. The "curtain" wall, built of insulated prefabricated panels of metal skins with insulation between, has been widely used, and when properly designed and constructed is trouble free. Moreover, it has the added advantage mentioned earlier of being easily removable for further expansion of the building, something which a masonry wall is not. Whatever type is used, it should be guaranteed weathertight for several years. The interior is usually "furred," or provided with a framework of small metal members, to support lath and plaster or some other material as an interior finish.

Partitions

Interior partitions, like the exterior walls, are also non-loadbearing, thus permitting them to be removed without affecting the structural support of the building. This flexibility can be increased, as previously mentioned, if they are made of steel studs carrying snap-in metal panels. The resulting finish is painted, and except for almost imperceptible joint lines, is as acceptable as a plastered wall. It has good sound-resisting qualities and can be fire-rated, something usually required of any hospital partition. They are thin, however, have limited capability in providing space for the runs of large pipes, and their flexibility is also curtailed by the fact that most of them will be enclosing plumbing pipes of some kind which must be rerouted or otherwise disposed of when the partition is removed. A somewhat more economical type of partition is the steel stud, rocklath, and plaster type which is currently in wide use throughout hospitals. It is also hollow, can be made wide enough to enclose most pipes, and its surface (plaster) can accept a variety of final finishes that can meet almost any requirement. In OR and similar rooms, this used to be ceramic tile, but unfortunately the joints in the latter are difficult to keep clean and have an alarming affinity for pathogens. Today a sprayed-on vitreous enamel finish is available which produces the same type surface as ceramic tile as a smooth surface without joints and is thus much easier to keep clean and bacteria-free. It is also much lower cost then ceramic tile. Other finishes available to be applied over plaster include tough vinyl wall coverings, resistant to mars and scratches and of pleasant soft appearance in a variety of colors and also easy to keep clean by washing; and a variety of paints, including spray-on vinyl paint and other coatings, with an astounding resistance to deterioration from scrubbing and which are relatively bacteriostatic. All such materials must be fire-resistant, a quality now determined by a rating called *flame-spread*. The term is from the Underwriters Laboratories testing procedures[*] which establish a flame-spread rating of 25 or less as a criterion for "incombustible."

Another type of partition available is the traditional masonry one. Composed of cinder or slag blocks four or six inches thick, it is usually finished in plaster applied directly to the

---

[*] American Society for Testing Materials No. E-84.

block and is thus capable of all the finishes that are applicable to plaster. It can also be finished with spray-on vitreous enamel directly over the block surface (producing an easily washable finish but one with the unevenness of the block and its joints) or it can be painted directly on the surface of the block. The latter finish is more advisable in the maintenance and utility areas of the hospital than the emergency department, however, since it is more difficult to keep clean and will often have pits and tiny indentations which could harbor bacteria. Moreover, it is almost impossible with "exposed block" to avoid some cracking due to the thermal stresses set up during the curing period and the seasonal expansion and contraction of the building. The latter is particularly true in a one-story structure. Such cracks, of course, have to be pointed and refinished, adding further woes to an already overburdened maintenance department.

Ceilings

The era of the hard, white plaster ceiling in hospitals is, happily, long since a thing of the past. In the emergency department, as in any patient care area, the ceiling should have three basic qualities: It should be easily removable, for access *anywhere* to the space above, which encloses a maze of pipes, conduits, and ducts; it should be extremely fire-resistant (a one-hour Underwriters' Laboratories fire rating is desirable, even if not always required), and it should be easily cleaned. In certain rooms and spaces where surgical procedures and trauma treatment will take place, it should have the same qualities of washability and freedom from compatibility with pathogens expected in the surgical suite. To this end, probably the most desirable material is aluminum acoustic tile, sound insulated, but without perforations. With a white baked-enamel finish, this comes about as close as possible to the ideal, but it is not the least expensive. Also available are panels of "lay-in" material, fiberglass or mineral, fissured or covered with various plastic smooth coatings, which are supported by a metal grid (2' × 2' or 2' × 4') of aluminum with or without a baked-on finish of enamel. These are less desirable in surgical or fracture rooms but serve well in spaces where the ultimate in asepsis is not a primary consideration. The panels can be raised and removed, permitting quick access to the utility passage space above, a highly desirable feature in our time when there seems to be constant necessity to add wiring or piping for some necessary change. A mineral-fiber acoustic board is available, at less cost than the metal pan-type referred to, which is described as "self-sanitizing" and is inhibitive to growth of bacteria.

Floors

The floor finishes applied in the emergency department—assuming that no flammable anesthetic agents will be permitted in any room—should generally be durable to heavy traffic, as nonslip as possible even when wet, easily cleanable by washing, and highly resistant to bacteria. To this end there should be, at least in surgical and fracture rooms and the open treatment area, no joints in the floor and a continuity without a break from the general floor to the top of a coved base. The ideal, of course, can never be quite attained, and those finishes which approach it are sadly the most expensive ones. There are, however, several trowelled-on floors available of epoxy, neoprene, and acrylic base which do an excellent job on all counts and come close to being bacteriostatic. They are available in the conductive form, designed for regular surgical suites where flammable anesthetics require this quality, but they are also available at less cost in a nonconductive type, well suited to the treatment areas of the emergency department. There is also an added advantage that a wider selection of more pleasant colors are available, whereas the conductive type is limited to plain black or a rather bleak black-and-white terrazzo. They are resistant to chemical staining or damage, are stable enough so that when properly installed no cracking can be expected, are relatively nonslip, and—with a high density—can easily be washed. Because of their relatively high cost, their use should be limited to areas where they are needed. If a conductive floor is used, be sure the conductivity is guaranteed to be permanent, without the use of saline solutions (it must comply with NFPA Standard No. 56-A). In spaces like the waiting and conference rooms, the most practical material, as in most locations, is the "resilient tile" that has become so ubiquitous, normally vinyl asbestos tile.

Windows

By far the best answer to the problem of what windows to use is *none*. Aside from the psychological problem of the occasional claustrophobic individual who must see the weather outside to be at ease, windows in the emergency department are simply a nuisance. Beyond that, they add to the air-conditioning load if the department has been blessed with summer cooling, and are an expensive maintenance problem to keep clean and undamaged. However, if windows there must be, the best approach is to reduce the nuisance to a minimum. Pivoted windows with single panes of glass that can be washed from the inside with a minimum of effort are achieving widespread acceptance in all parts of hospitals, and they would appear the best to use here. It should be remembered, however, that if there are windows in observation rooms where psychotic patients may be held for even a short time, the window glass should be the tempered type which cannot be broken under normal circumstances. Also, window hardware should be such that permits only one window in a room to be opened by an occupant a few inches, so that disturbed patients cannot open one wide enough to permit passage of their bodies. (The pivoting for cleaning purposes is controlled by a key kept elsewhere.)

Doors

The entrance door to the department for trauma patients, usually brought by ambulance or other vehicle, will hopefully have been located under a wide enough canopy to permit at least two ambulances to unload simultaneously. Since the patients are being brought in by stretcher, often with an attendant walking alongside holding an I.V. bottle, the entrance (as mentioned in Chapter 2) will be wide enough to permit such entrance without delay and without causing *additional* trauma. Usually a pair of doors will be required, and if possible these should open automatically. There are two types of such doors available, one of which slides apart with each half of the door recessing into a slot at the sides. This, of course, requires the entrance passage to be wide enough to accept the sliding doors when open. The swing type operate normally, swinging into the department when electrically activated by foot pad, push button, or photoelectric cell, as are the sliding type. Most applicable building codes require all exit doors to swing out as a fire requirement. Both types of doors are available with a device that permits them to be swung open on hinges when pushed from the inside, in which case they swing out, thus satisfying the code requirements. Probably the foot-pad type of operation is the most desirable, since ambulance attendants do not have to look for a push button, and the pad provides a nonslip surface at the entrance to prevent falls. The pad (as stated in Chapter 2) can be recessed to avoid a tripping hazard. Vestibules are highly desirable to prevent arctic blasts inside during winter weather but should be deep enough to permit easy passage.

Interior doors should be—as should most doors in the hospital for negotiation by stretcher—wide enough to permit access under the conditions which can be expected. Normally, this is a minimum of four feet, but if fracture-room doors are to permit the passage of stretchers with patients in traction, even wider access should be considered. Hardware for treatment-room doors can be the convenient type operated by elbow or wrist by a nurse carrying a tray or other equipment. If holding or observation rooms are included, it may be desirable to have hardware only on the outside to prevent a disturbed patient from opening the door from the inside or damaging himself on the knob. All doors where stretchers or carts must pass should be protected by "armor-plating," a tough plastic covering over the door from the bottom to a height above the top of such vehicles. Other doors are best protected by kickplates, a plastic strip at the bottom only. The incredible amount of damage done by stretchers to unprotected doors of a recently completed surgical suite visited by the writer is ample proof of the value of such protection. One wonders what happened to the patients during the many collisions.

Casework

Aside from the question of durability and quality, the main problem with casework is to get an adequate amount but not an over supply. When you open a wall cabinet in a utility room and find nothing but the nurses' luncheon bags and pocketbooks, the hospital has thrown money away on expensive equipment because someone did not do his homework. The storage problem needs to be studied in adequate detail to determine where various articles will be placed and to ensure enough space is provided to take care of the need. Either too much or too little is unsatisfactory. Most casework is steel with baked enamel finish, although some surgical rooms are equipped with all stainless steel cabinets or with baked enamel cabinets having stainless steel shelves and door and drawer fronts.

Communications

Communication systems in the emergency department can vary widely in their degree of sophistication, and thus their cost. As a minimum, there should be telephonic communication with the hospital switchboard as a means of alerting doctors on call for emergency service. When the hospital has an interior dial system or an interdepartmental "intercom" system, vital communication with other departments of the hospital is facilitated. The relative advantages of the two systems do not find universal agreement,[2] but whatever system is available should make quick and easy communication possible without long waits between the emergency department and laboratories, radiology, the surgical suite, medical records, central sterile supply, pharmacy, intensive care, and administration. At least one phone with a direct outside line is essential. In addition, there should be at least two pay phones available for the waiting room, and a conference room or other space usable by police should be equipped for making outside phone calls. Intercommunication by a local system within the department should provide for "hands off" voice communication between all closed-treatment and surgery and fracture rooms with the nurses' station, and a nurses' call system (preferably by voice) should connect the nurses' station with observation beds and patients' beds in the open-cubicle treatment area. In fact, some codes require this. There should be a call-registering light over the door or access to each patient's bed or bedroom.

There should be a bell button with call-registering light at the outside entrance door to the department, so that late arriving patients can signal the reception desk or nurses' station. This is particularly true in hospitals where the door must be kept locked for security at certain hours.

A recent innovation in emergency department communications worthy of careful consideration in new construction because of its potential in saving lives is radio communication with ambulances while enroute to the hospital. Such a two-way radio net should also be extended to include local police nets. With a system of this type in operation, it is possible for the police or ambulance crew to alert the emergency department well before arrival to the apparent nature and extent of injuries in accident cases, the number of patients to be expected, etc., so that preparations may be well under way long before the ambulance rolls up to the entrance door. In cases of coronary attack or infarctions, where minutes count in the saving of lives, the system will make it possible for the "crash team" to be waiting at the door, equipment and drugs ready. Some hospitals, anticipating the more remote possibility of catastrophic disaster conditions, have installed such radio communications to include state police and the nearest two or three hospitals capable of handling major emergency cases, so that communications are available in the event the local telephone lines are nonfunctioning. In the event that any such radio communication is installed, regardless of the degree, it is of course essential that the power supply for it be part of the emergency power system of the hospital in anticipation of the possibility that normal power sources may also be nonoperative.

In addition to normal voice communication between the emergency department and other ancillary areas upon which it depends, a valuable additional system is the pneumatic tube, which in the last few years has come of age to the degree that it has vastly improved (electronic) controls and generally trouble-free performance. The speed with which it can transport supplies, specimens, drugs, films, reports, medical records, and written messages between remote parts of the building makes it highly worthy of consideration. Its rather high initial cost at installation should be carefully weighed against the savings it can effect over a long period of time in manpower.

Mechanical, Plumbing

The plumbing systems in the emergency department have to do with hot and cold water, oxygen and suction lines, medical gases (if any), compressed air (if any), and the various fixtures served by these systems. The normal water closets and sinks or lavatories are typical throughout the hospital and hardly need discussion, other than to state that by far the best type of toilet, from the maintenance standpoint, is the "wall-hung" variety, which permits easy cleaning of the floor around and under it. All handwashing type sinks, including regular toilet rooms, should be equipped with wrist-type operating trim, and of course those provided in surgical or fracture or treatment rooms should be suitable to the scrubbing process and supplied with the approved type of liquid antiseptic soap. The soiled utility room should have a "clinical" sink, usually referred to by the nursing staff as a "flushing rim" sink, in addition to a normal lavatory-type sink. The latter can be a stainless steel counter sink. The use of a bedpan sterilizer in utility rooms is generally considered a thing of the past, since clinical sinks or toilets can be equipped with bedpan washers, and all bedpans should go to Central Sterile Supply for decontamination and autoclaving after their use by a single patient is concluded. The use of disposable bedpans, urinals, and emesis basins is becoming more and more widespread, which also contributes to the passing of the bedpan sterilizer. Clinical sinks should be mounted on a base to avoid having to bend over when using them.

Outlets for oxygen and suction can be mounted in a console over the head of the bed or table, combined with the light, in an observation bedroom or treatment room or alcove, or in a wall panel near the head. There are several manufacturers who can supply relatively foolproof outlet units provided with safety valves, and care should be taken to see that whatever brand is supplied is one of tried and established reputation. The same applies to medical gas-dispensing outlets, if they are used.

When plumbing fixtures are selected, they must meet specific requirements of the federal and possibly other codes in their design.

Mechanical, Heating, Ventilating, and Air-conditioning

"Ventilation of the emergency department should provide fresh air at comfortable temperatures and should avoid the dissemination of infection. Air conditioning is desirable; the system should incorporate temperature and humidity control and adequate filtration or precipitation to eliminate dissemination of bacteria-laden dust."[3,p30] The system, to accomplish these highly desirable goals, can be designed in many degrees of sophistication. As a minimum, the desirable parameters of temperature range, relative humidity range, and air changes per hour should be maintained. Beyond that, it is desirable to approach the condition of maximum asepsis, particularly in closed surgical and fracture rooms, by producing a higher pressure within the room than without, supplying 100 percent outside air, and not recirculating air in the rooms where asepsis is desired, at least during use. Exhausts near the floor are desirable to remove dust and medical gases, which are heavier than air and linger near the floor. A new system of air supply and exhaust to operating rooms, called *Laminar Flow,* is coming into use, and may become applicable on the basis of the dictum stated in Chapter 2 that treatment rooms in emergency should achieve a condition of asepsis comparable to that in the surgical suite, to certain rooms in emergency. It consists of air supplied through a large area under very heavy pressure and in great volume, carefully filtered, and it is intended to produce optimum conditions in the reduction of air-borne pathogens.

In designing the "HVAC" systems, the engineer must pay particular attention to the requirements of the governing codes. The current *General Standards of Construction and Equipment for Hospitals and Medical Facilities* of the Federal Public Health Service, which governs all Hill-Burton assisted projects and controls most others, is very specific about the volume of air supplied to various type rooms and whether it can be recirculated or not. It requires emergency operating rooms, for example, to have five minimum changes of outdoor air per hour, twelve minimum total air changes per hour, a positive pressure relationship to adjacent areas, and it permits no recirculation of air within the room. These requirements, incidentally, are exactly those for operating rooms in the surgical suite. Isolation rooms, which may house contaminated patients, also have stringent requirements.

The usual method—and probably the most efficient for normal use—of air supply is by means of the ceiling "diffuser," the visible round or square louvered-ceiling outlet. It distributes the air as desired but has the disadvantage of requiring not infrequent cleaning to remove dust particles that tend to adhere to its periphery. Diffusers are sometimes equipped with hard surfaced plastic dust rings intended to separate the fixture from ceiling tiles of porous material more likely to collect the dust.

Another system recently developed for the transmission of air is the ventilating troffer, a light fixture designed to supply air from openings around its rim. This fixture is desirable from the standpoint that, when usable, it eliminates what is often a conflict in design between lights and diffusers for the available space in a ceiling, but the volume of air supplied is much less than from diffusers, and often it simply will not supply enough.

As important as the design and installation of the heating and ventilating and air-conditioning systems is the final balancing after completion. If the building is equipped with air-conditioning (summer cooling) and is completed in the winter, the contractor is required as part of his contract to return and balance the cooling system when outside temperatures warrant the use of its cooling cycle. Until this has been accomplished, the best system that can be built will not work properly and will overcool in one area and leave the occupants sweltering in another. The reverse is equally true, of course, for the heating cycle. The controls over the system, which involve complexities that are wisely left to the tender care of the competent maintenance department, are usually the last part of the system to be put in working order, and also take a period of adjustment which is part of the "balancing" act. Until all of the various components have been approved by the engineer, some patience is usually necessary on the part of the occupying staff; but this does not preclude the reporting of trouble as it occurs, since the best criterion of a balanced system is the comfort of all the human beings who occupy it.

Electrical

In considering the electrical work that goes into an emergency department, three major items need to be considered: lighting, power, and electrical hazards. Lighting will generally be of the recessed fluorescent luminaire type, with fixtures four feet long and of various widths, to obtain general illumination of a minimum of 100 footcandles throughout the area, with more intense and special lights in specific places for specific purposes. Operating and fracture rooms should usually have a capacity of 2000 footcandles, with adjustable levels up to that point. The type of tubes used in the fluorescent fixtures should be such that will be as near to daylight as possible, neither color accentuating or color deficient. Special examining lights for treatment areas can be obtained with quartz sources that provide high-intensity illumination, with retracting arms permitting them to be focused on any part of the patient. Such lights have the disadvantage of producing high heat intensity along with the excellent quality of the illumination, and cannot be held close to a patient's skin for too long. Portable examining lights on stands or supported on I.V. poles are available also.

An adequate number of x-ray viewing boxes should be provided in strategic locations throughout the department, including, of course, a battery of several in a fracture room or surgical treatment room. They can be either recessed or surface mounted.

In order to be certain that lighting fixtures have been thoroughly understood, it is customary for the electrical engineer to show a catalogue of cuts or drawings and/or photographs of all individual types of lighting fixtures for approval. It should be made clear at the time of submission of such a brochure what controls are available and where they will be located. If dimming of lights at night is required, it is possible to obtain dimming control of the fluorescent fixtures at a considerable cost. Another and less expensive method of dimming is to switch several circuits of lights separately, so that alternate fixtures, for example, can be separately extinguished, thus reducing the illumination. The best type of cover over the fluorescent tubes is the plastic lens type, easily removable by releasing hinges, for replacement of tubes. The "eggcrate" type of cover is not advisable, because of its tendency to permit dust to accumulate within the fixture and then drop below.

Electrical power for emergency department "must be adequate and available through enough outlets to provide for the operation of all lights and equipment at a maximum utilization."[3,p31] Since the emergency department will probably be at its peak use in periods when natural conditions or manmade catastrophies have eliminated the normal power supply, it should have all of its outlets powered by the hospital's emergency standby power source, including all special outlets of higher voltage for special equipment, such as 220-volt receptacles for portable x-ray, and all powered equipment in surgical and fracture rooms. For such rooms, the operating room electrical facility panels, which provide operating room circuits properly grounded, protected against electrical leakage hazards, and protected by isolating transformers, are a highly desirable feature. Such isolating transformers should also be available to a cardiac treatment room, if one is to be used, since the possibility of electrical shock adequate enough to cause fibrillation is most likely to occur to a patient with external transducers applied and an internal pacemaker being installed (see chapter on equipment). Adequate grounding of all circuits within the department is essential, through proper three-prong receptacles and protection against electrical leakage. (This is further stressed in Chapter 16 in discussion of the equipment in the cardiac receiving room.)

CONTRACT DOCUMENT PHASE

The "contract document" phase of his work is the only one in which the architect and his engineers prepare the actual drawings and specifications which the building contractors use to construct the project. Since they are technical documents intended for the use of specialists in the technology of building construction, they are no longer made as a means of explaining a complicated idea to a group of individuals untrained in this field, and they are therefore extremely difficult for others to read and understand. This is particularly true with hospital documents, involving as they do highly detailed dimensional layouts of rooms and spaces and just about all the mechanical and electrical systems that are possible to combine in one structure. The working drawings for a $15 million major hospital expansion program today can easily number 150 sheets of drawings approximately 36″ by 48″ in size, and the specifications 1000 or more pages of double-spaced type. Naturally, only a portion of these would be concerned with the emergency department, but the difficulty of absorbing all of the information conveyed, even for a limited section of the building, is a formidable one.

Nevertheless, the time-consuming chore of sitting down and listening and questioning while they are explained is as important as the initial planning. It is the only way to ensure that the dimensions will permit equipment and carts to pass through doors and passages; that the floor, wall, and ceiling finishes are proper for aseptic and sanitary conditions as well as ease of maintenance; that lighting is adequate for the purpose of each space; that plumbing and ventilation are to do the job; and that equipment is the right type and will be in the right place to perform its function in the best possible way.

Moreover, this review is perhaps the most important of all for the very considerable reason that it is the final one. After this, the only way to revise is by changing a legal contract, which generally results in a delay and an exorbitant increase in cost, factors that cause administrators and trustee committees to regard the belated requests for such changes with an extremely jaundiced eye.

There are many drawings and specifications involved in the project at this time which need not concern the committee. Those involving structural elements and how they are constructed, except insofar as they affect space utilization or ceiling heights, are best left to the engineer. So also are those details required for the construction of exterior walls, mechanical and utility areas, piping riser diagrams, mechanical details, and many others of the purely technical variety. Those which should be reviewed are the floor plans, including the large-scale detailed plans of special areas, such as OR, nurses' station, or utility room; the reflected ceiling plans, which show the location of lights, ventilating diffusers, etc.; the finishes, usually described on a "schedule of finishes"; door sizes, shown on a "door schedule"; mechanical plans, which show the locations of oxygen and suction and medical gases, if any, as well as plumbing fixtures; elevation drawings, which show such exterior details as a canopy for ambulances to unload under weather protection; and those detail drawings of architectural, mechanical, and electrical sections which show the type of special equipment to be built in at various locations, such as casework (wall and base cabinets, counters and sinks), OR electrical facility panels, lights, scrub sinks, clocks, film illuminators (view boxes), outlet locations for portable x-ray machines (or permanently installed ones in OR's or fracture rooms); telephone and intercom system equipment; examining lights; sphygmomanometer locations; monitoring equipment, such as EKG oscilloscopes, if one or more is to be permanently installed in a cardiac treatment room; and all the other myriad of devices, equipment, outlets, and facilities that have to do with the actual medical use of the various rooms and spaces.

A checklist is an excellent assist in reviewing the final drawings. Probably even better would be for selected individuals from the various staff sections concerned with emergency to spend enough time looking at them to be able to project themselves into the plan as they will later actually use the facility. This takes imagination and concentration, but if the trained medical mind can see itself actually treating a patient in a given space, actually using the light, applying the oxygen mask, reading the monitor, taking the x-ray, suturing the wound, treating the burns, antidoting the poison, administering the tranquilizer to a disturbed mental patient, deciding what to do next when four trauma cases arrive simultaneously, it will be time worth spending, for it will reveal before it is too late those oversights that can be corrected, those situations which require something arranged a little differently for greater efficiency. This must be done with the developed drawings alongside—for only they will show movable furniture in place, or tables, and so forth.

The contract specifications generally serve to augment and refine the information given on the contract drawings, describing the quality of an item shown on the drawings or the type of performance expected from a given piece of equipment. Some portions may be written as a "closed" specification; that is, the item is named by a brand as being required under the contract, so no performance data is required. When it can be avoided, this system is less desirable than naming two or three brands, all of which are considered acceptable, or by specifying a performance standard. Both the latter two types encourage competitive bidding and thereby lower costs. The important thing for the committee is to be sure that the "closed" brand, or the three brands, or the performance represents what is known and desired. To ensure this, it will often be necessary for staff members to have visited other hospitals to inspect the item and actually see it in use, a process sometimes difficult to impose upon busy doctors, nurses, and administrators. The educational process necessary to convince people that hospital equipment may have improved in the last ten or twenty years can be a surprisingly difficult one at times, but is quite essential if an institution is to maintain the high standards of perform-ance that will enable it to survive and grow.

The costs of all the components of the building, something which cannot have been allowed to be forgotten throughout the various steps the project has undergone, are even more im-portant at this stage, because when the contract documents are approved they will shortly be a hard fact of life when bids are received. And the cost of quality, as always, is high. Be-cause of this, and because the bidding process is an unpre-dictable one subject to the vagaries of the economy, the time of year, the political and international situations, and many social and industrial unknowns, the specifications will probably include a number of alternate proposals. These are deletions, substitutions, or additions to the basic specifications intended to reveal, in actual dollar costs, what such a change would mean to the budget. An alternate proposal may be included for one of three reasons: To determine the cost of something desired, but not included in the project budget, thus permitting its in-clusion if bids are received below estimates; to determine the price of certain items which could be eliminated if the bids come in too high for the pocketbook; or to provide a com-petitive product in order to offset a "closed" specification, thus encouraging a lower bid. The owner has the option, at the time bids are received, to accept or reject any alternate, and he thus retains some flexibility in the establishment of the ultimate con-tract amount.

Another part of the specifications, called "general conditions" lists various requirements designed to protect an owner against the many legal pitfalls and entrapments inherent in all con-tracts. These, however, are more properly the province of the hospital's attorneys than of the building committee.

One aspect of the specifications that may be included, how-ever, can be of extreme importance to the committee. If the project is an addition and/or alteration to an existing building, the detailed sequence of the actual construction operation is often spelled out as a contract requirement, in order to ensure the uninterrupted day-to-day use of existing facilities while the work is going on. This aspect of building operations in hospitals is one of the most difficult problems to resolve, and one which, if improperly handled, can create havoc. Since the building process itself is by its very nature a dirty, dusty, noisy, and thoroughly unpleasant environment, to have it going on even near a hospital is unfortunate, but if it is proceeding inside a hospital, it introduces conditions which are the antithesis of everything a hospital represents and strives to obtain. Taken at its best it is a difficult, antitherapeutic, and highly annoying necessity with which a staff can ruefully live in the expectation of the great day in the future when the new facility will be opened for use, but at its worst it can create confusion and upheavals that not only tear apart the patient care process but cause temper-shattering rifts between staff and administration and even threaten mass resignations. The solution, of course, is once more intelligent foresight and careful planning. The resultant "procedure of construction" or "sequence of operations" may necessarily cost the hospital more dollars than normal construction, since at the very least it may require certain work to be done at night or on weekends at greatly increased labor rates. In the emergency department, if it is open on a 24-hour basis, it may be extremely difficult to work out an acceptable scheme. Some of the measures which can be taken to ease the pain include the use of temporary dustproof partitions, carefully sealed with tape and perhaps even sound insulated, between construction areas and those remaining in use by the hospital. The extending of utility pipes and electrical facilities can be expedited by constructing the extension and then turning off the utility for a very brief period to make final connections at a time least likely to cause harmful effects, such as between three and five o'clock in the morning. To protect against unexpected problems, standby facilities can be held ready. For example, if oxygen lines must be on "down time" for a certain period, portable equipment in adequate amounts must be available on call. A switchover to emergency electric power can often fill the gap when the main power service is temporarily inactivated. All such problems must be carefully thought out, and plans must be made for the unexpected contingency situation. In the emergency department, fervent prayers are often added that a major influx of trauma patients from unexpected highway or other disasters will not occur during the inactivation of much needed utilities.

Such a "procedure of construction" will be extremely important if new construction of ancillary service areas combines with a reassignment of existing facilities to new purposes—for example, when the emergency department moves into new quarters, and for example, laboratories expand into space previously occupied by emergency. Obviously, with such moves depending on sequential preparation of areas to keep all departments in operation without interruption, new facilities must be completed and occupied before alteration work to change the existing spaces can be undertaken.

REFERENCES

1. Fitzimmons, Robert J.: *Facts and Trends in Hospital Outpatient Services.* PHS Publication No. 930-C-6.
2. Schwartz, Lawrence: Intercoms relieve overworked telephones. *Mod Hosp, 116:4,* pp. 92–93, 1971.
3. *The Emergency Department in the Hospital: A Guide to Organization and Management.* Chicago, American Hospital Association, 1962, p. 30.

Chapter 5

EQUIPMENT

The equipment for any department of a hospital should be selected by those who are to use it. The two lists presented here are merely suggestions which may be used as guides, additions or subtractions being made by the medical staff. The items listed will equip the department for care of most emergencies. The first list includes large articles of furniture as well as items of professional equipment; the second, smaller items, practically all for professional use. Those needed for prompt use are listed as sets or packs, and it is suggested that these be assembled, sterilized, and clearly marked. Labeling is of major importance as no one can be expected to recognize these packs from their shape. Some hospitals find it advantageous to wrap lifesaving packs, such as tracheostomy sets, in distinctive colored wrappers. Tongue depressors, shellacked and lettered with India ink, make good markers. These should be put on each pack in central supply or wherever the sets are sterilized. All cabinets and drawers in which they are stored should also be labeled as to contents.

It cannot be repeated too often that all the equipment should be purchased for and belong to the emergency department, to be used there only. The department should not borrow or loan, except for very special items of equipment. No discards from other departments should be used.

Most of the items listed are well known to those who will use them. A few will be discussed in detail with the hope that this will be helpful in selecting the most usable equipment. The contents of some of the sterile packs are itemized, but it should be clearly understood that the articles for these in any department should be selected in accordance with the wishes of the doctors who will use the sets.

THE BIG THINGS

Stretchers.
Wheelchairs.
Resuscitation equipment.
Oxygen tanks with reduction valves.
Anesthesia equipment (gases and oxygen may be piped in).
Suction machine, unless wall suction is available.
Cardiac pacemaker.
Defibrillator.
Portable floor lights.
Portable x-ray, unless built into the fracture room.
Standards for intravenous solutions.
Kick buckets on castors.
Mayo stands.
Basin stands.
Operating table if operating room is provided.
Refrigerator.
Desk or table.
Straight-back chairs.
Stools.
File cabinet.

THE SMALLER THINGS

Emergency sets or packs.
    Tracheostomy.
    Thoracotomy.
    Thoracostomy.
    Catheterization.
    Obstetrical.
    Wound irrigation.
    Wound debridement and suture.
    Minor wound suture.
    Gastric lavage.
    Lumbar puncture.
    Paracentesis.
    Venesection.
    Blood culture.
Splints
    Thomas or Keller-Blake.
    Coaptation—wood or aluminum.
    Pneumatic, if approved by staff.
    Cervical collars.

Sphygmomanometers—on wall, and portable.
Stethoscopes.
Airways.
Flashlights.
Otoscope.
Ophthalmoscope.
Nasal specula.
Vaginal specula.
Bedpans.
Basins and trays.
Surgeon's gloves.
Syringes.
    Asepto.
    Luer Type—2 cc, 5 cc, 10 cc, 20 cc, 30 cc, and 50 cc.
Hypodermic needles.
    Assorted sizes and lengths.
Cast cutter.
Surgical instruments.
    Hemostats—large and small.
    Needle holders.
    Suture needles.
    Tissue forceps.
    Sponge forceps.
    Scissors—straight and curved.
Books and manuals.
    American College of Surgeons manuals.
      An Outline of the Treatment of Fractures—1965.
      Early Care of Soft Tissue Injuries—1965.
    Textbooks of medicine, surgery, anatomy, physiology, pediatrics, and microbiology.
    Poison manual or toxicology textbook, card index of poisons and antidotes.

Stretchers

Stretchers* should be the type designed for emergency department or recovery room use. They should be capable of being put in Trendelenburg or reverse Trendelenburg positions, preferably with crank handles. They should have racks for oxygen tanks, removable standards at either end for intravenous solutions, arm boards, and easily adjustable side rails.

* The emergency department stretcher is not only for transportation; it is the treatment table, and patients should be shifted as infrequently as possible.

A built-in mechanism for raising or lowering the height should be provided. Provision for elevating the head and shoulders of orthopneic patients should be a feature. Examples of these are shown in Figures 32 and 33. Such tables are expensive; they will cost $500 to $1000 with all the accessories. It does not pay to economize on these, as they will be subject to constant and sometimes rough usage.

The casters of the stretchers should be large (8 inch) and capable of being locked at both ends. These stretchers will be used to transport patients into the x-ray department, to the operating room, and to the wards and patients' rooms, and small casters are not satisfactory. To ensure a degree of com-

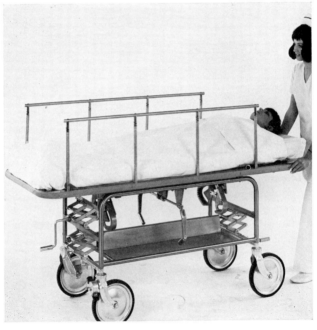

Figure 32A

Figure 32. *A*, Hausted-Simmons Easy-Lift stretcher. Shows large conductive swivel casters with locks, retracting side rails, intravenous rod, height adjustment crank, Fowler and Trendelenburg positioning, and two-way slide and tilt-top. *B*, Hausted-Simmons Easy-Lift stretcher with slide and tilt-top being used to transfer patient to bed. *C*, Hausted-Simmons Conver-Table showing adjustment for Gyn and Fowler positions.

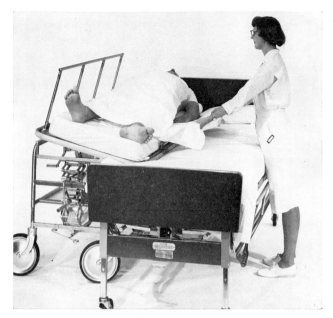

Figure 32B

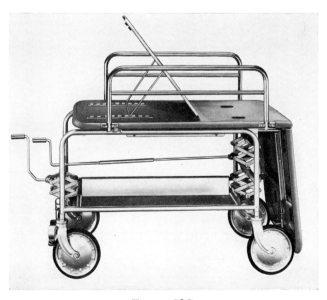

Figure 32C

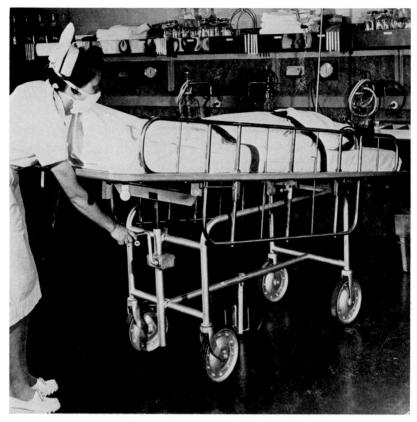

Figure 33. Jarvis and Jarvis stretcher. Shows large casters, crank elevator, side rails, intravenous rod, and Trendelenburg positioning.

fort when patients have to remain on the stretchers for some time, the stretchers should have pads three or four inches thick, covered with plastic or rubberized material. If these pads are x-ray translucent, they will allow the technicians to slide cassettes under them, making a shift of the patient to the x-ray table unnecessary (see Figs. 32A and 33).

Stretchers so constructed that they can slide over an x-ray table without shifting the patient have real advantages. The author has seen one of these, the *Surgilift*, shown in Figures 34A and 34B in use and highly recommended by those using it. Another is the Transaver, a removable litter used on a low cart (the Shuttler) (see Fig. 35A), by ambulance crews and on

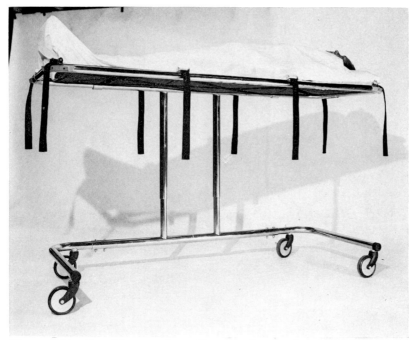

Figure 34A. Surgilift stretcher. Shows radio-translucent material rein-
forced with webbing straps.

a high cart (the Straddler) (see Fig. 35B), in hospitals.
The legs of the high cart swing out for straddling the x-ray
table, or in for transportation within the hospital. Figure 35C
shows it over a conventional emergency department stretcher,
in this case the Stryker. The Stryker is a first-class stretcher
with which the author has had experience. It has an unusual
collection of useful accessories. The Transaver also has a Fowler
backpiece and Trendelenburg position attachment, as well as
side rails and an IV mast. Either of these stretchers will limit
the number of times a patient is moved.

Wheelchairs

Wheelchairs should not be the old wooden variety that
occupied so much space and tipped over at the least provocation.
For decades, the wheelchair and the bedpan were probably the

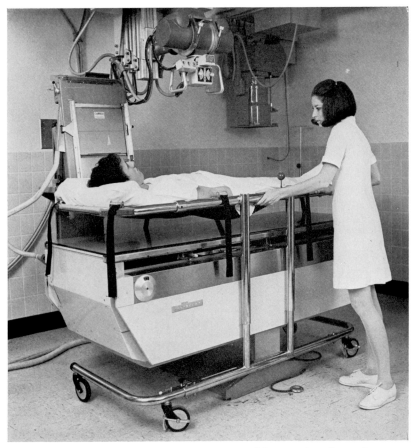

Figure 34B. Surgilift stretcher over an x-ray table. Height of stretcher may be adjusted.

pieces of hospital equipment most neglected by designers. Now, some degree of comfort is provided in both, and their hazards have been decreased. Well-built folding wheelchairs are available that will occupy much less space, when not in use, than the old type.

Resuscitation Equipment

Although mechanical, positive-pressure resuscitation was first introduced in 1927, it was not until 15 years later that

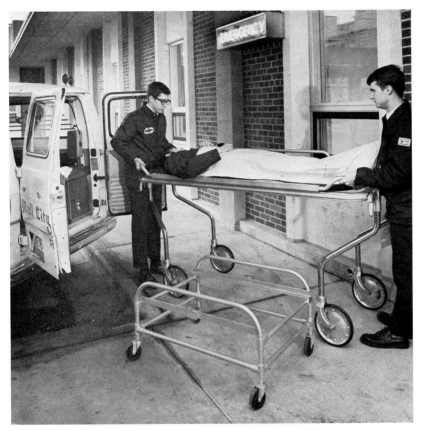

Figure 35A. Transaver stretcher. Photograph shows the "Shuttler" (the low ambulance cart) and the "Straddler" onto which the patient has just been placed without being moved from the stretcher. The Straddler is for use in the hospital.

the Council on Physical Medicine of the American Medical Association gave its approval. Authorities who resisted approval during the thirties were concerned with possible lung damage from too much pressure. They continued to advocate a simple inhalation apparatus, such as that designed by Henderson and Haggard in 1920. This was useless unless the patient was breathing, so had to be accompanied by manual artificial respiration. There is little doubt that the application of the prone pressure or other types of artificial respiration to patients with certain types of injuries was more dangerous than the use of

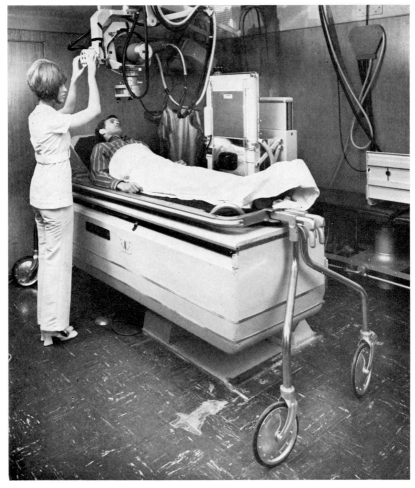

Figure 35B. Transaver Straddler, with legs swung out to straddle the x-ray table.

automatic pressure-controlled respiration. This equipment, if of the alternate positive and negative pressure type, provides four ounces of positive pressure per square inch and three ounces negative pressure. With this lesser amount of negative pressure, all the air is not withdrawn from the lungs. The respiratory rate, when this apparatus is in use, automatically adjusts to the lung capacity in patients from adults to infants.

The apparatus provides a signal if the airway is clogged.

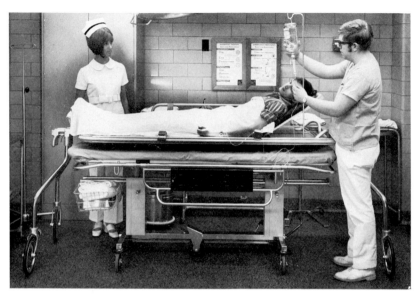

Figure 35C. Transaver Straddler showing intravenous standard and head elevator. Here the Transaver straddles another good stretcher, the Stryker. The Stryker has a good set of useful accessories, including retracting side rails and a stretcher frame that may be lifted off the carriage to avoid extra moves of the patient.

This is a rapid clicking of the machine. This, plus no evidence of chest expansion, signals the need for clearing the airway. If the obstruction is mucus or other liquid, a suction tip is inserted into the pharynx, and the machine is switched to suction by moving a small lever. This is a simple procedure and requires only a moment. If solids, such as pieces of undigested food are present, manual clearing of the airway will be required. Occasionally, all that is needed to provide a free airway is a change of position of the head and neck.

As recovery takes place, the rhythmic clicking of the machine at the end of the respiratory cycle will become irregular. This signals the return of physiologic respirations, and the lever may be switched to inhalation. There are several models of alternating pressure machines available.

One model of resuscitator, the *Bird Mark 17 Volume Limiting Respirator*, provides no negative pressure. This allows expiration to take place as the result of pressure in the chest. This model is favored by some authorities. This machine is also provided with suction and may be used as an inhalator when respiration is resumed naturally.

The widespread use of these positive-pressure machines indicates their almost universal approval. This is truly lifesaving equipment. There are sound arguments against the use of these by poorly trained rescue squads, although many lay first-aid and rescue workers have mastered them. There is every reason to use them in emergency departments with trained personnel. There is further discussion on this subject later in this chapter under *Equipment Hazards.*

High insufflation pressures to attain sufficient alveolar ventilation may cause leakage between the mask and the face. This is not dangerous, but it does decrease the effectiveness of the treatment. Hedstrand[1] studied different resuscitators and points out that difficult anatomical conditions of the face, as in elderly people, or inability of the operator to hold the mask on tightly may be factors in this leakage. It is much less likely to occur if the operator is able to use both hands.

After discussing at some length the features of various resuscitators made in Sweden, Hedstrand states, "The main conclusion drawn from the described tests is that the way in which good types of resuscitators are used—i.e. the skill in performing artificial ventilation in patients with lung airway resistance—is of more importance than details in their design." This simply reemphasizes the statement made by the author in various chapters in this book, that the training and experience of the personnel is the most important feature in planning for good emergency department care.

It hardly seems necessary to point out that these resuscitators are not applicable when external cardiac compression is being administered, but there are many emergency situations in which cardiac action is present but respiration is not. Here the resuscitator proves its worth when properly used.

Oxygen Tanks

Oxygen tanks are combined with the resuscitation apparatus, but separate tanks with reduction valves and face masks will prove valuable for patients who, due to shallow breathing or other reasons, need a higher concentration of oxygen than available in room air. This equipment also calls for frequent inspection to assure competent valves and full tanks.

Hand-operated resuscitators are easy to use, economical, and almost foolproof. Their use is easy to teach to personnel, and almost no time is lost in activating them. Health Devices[2] lists three of these as "acceptable" (Fig. 36, A, B and C). The Laerdal, model RFB-11, has three sizes of transparent masks. The Puritan, model PMR, also has a transparent mask. The Ambu, which is used by the U.S. Armed Forces and many of the NATO armed forces, should be obtained with a transparent mask so that vomitus entering the mask may be seen. Pur-

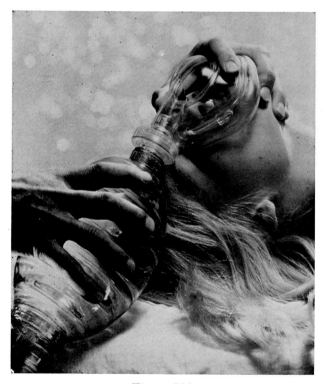

Figure 36A

Figure 36. Hand-operated resuscitators. A, Laerdal, Model RFB-11. B, Puritan, Model PMR. C, Ambu with foot pump for suction.

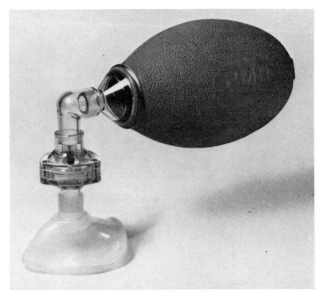

Figure 36B

chasers should be sure that they obtain the type with the E-2 valve, as it eliminates some problems connected with the older type valve. The Ambu may be operated with a foot pump, seen in the illustration. This will aid in removing vomitus and tracheal or pharyngeal secretions, but it must not be depended on to remove solid material in vomitus. Such material has to be removed manually, regardless of the apparatus being used.

Anesthesia Equipment

As stated elsewhere, there are varying opinions regarding the use of *general inhalation anesthesia* in emergency departments. These opinions are sometimes based on an experience limited to a particular hospital or type of hospital. It would be wrong to generalize on which opinion is correct. If trained personnel is available, all necessary equipment up to standard, the environment favorable, and proper attention given to preoperative preparation, patients may be safely anesthetized here. One thing, however, must be assured; anesthesia machines and resuscitators should belong to this department and not be

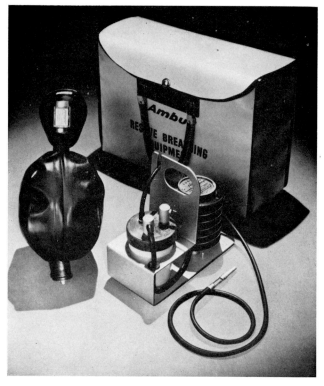

Figure 36C

shared with the operating room suite. The transfer of this equipment back and forth will divide the responsibility for its proper maintenance and sooner or later lead to dangerous breakdowns in service. This equipment should remain under the authority of the department of anesthesiology even though it may be budgeted by the emergency department. If the hospital is small and does not have an organized department of anesthesiology, general anesthesia should not be used outside of the operating and delivery rooms. It would be safer to transfer patients needing this service to the operating room where they will be in the hands of anesthetists accustomed to working there.

Equipment for *intravenous anesthesia* is simple and easy to keep in order. An adequate supply of syringes, needles, and tubing should be on hand as well as the anesthetic media and supportive drugs used by the anesthetists. Intravenous anesthesia used here should be of the safest types, and long anesthetic procedures should be discouraged. Unusual relaxation is rarely needed in emergency room surgical procedures and the various muscle-relaxing agents are better not used. Resuscitation equipment in good order is mandatory for the rare case of respiratory paralysis. A suction machine or wall suction must be provided.

No one can object to *local anesthesia*. The big problem is to get all the staff to use it when indicated. Sessions devoted to instruction in local anesthesia techniques would be valuable in many hospitals, particularly for physicians practicing in the emergency department.

A variety of 2, 5, 10, and 20 cc syringes in individual sterile packs should be available, as well as *sharp* needles, particularly 20, 21, and 22 gauge, in 1, 1½, and 2-inch lengths.

Emergency Sets

Tracheostomy: Scalpel handle and blades of the type approved by the staff, small hemostats, skin hooks, small retractors, plain gut and silk (000 or 0000), sutures with curved cutting-edge needles, needle holder, and a variety of tracheostomy tubes. In the last few years, these tubes have been improved by having a more truly anatomic curve. There is also a tube with an inflatable rubber cuff. Gauze squares and tape to keep the tube in place complete the set.

Thoracotomy: For open cardiac massage. Dissection set and rib-spread retractor.

Thoracostomy: Scalpel with small blade, Foley catheters for intercostal drainage, and bottles and tubing for underwater seal drainage.

Wound Irrigation: In spite of the admonition of the thirties to use "gallons and gallons" of water in irrigating wounds, this much is seldom required. For large wounds, a flask with long rubber tubing and a glass tip should be ready in a sterile set. For small wounds, irrigation with saline solution injected from a large Asepto syringe is quite satisfactory. In this set should be a basin for the sterile saline solution, a sponge forceps, and some gauze squares. The removal of small foreign bodies, such as cinders and gravel, can often be aided by sponging while the wound is being irrigated.

Wound Debridement and Suture Set: The presence on a suture tray of instruments for debridement will always be appreciated by the doctor experienced in wound care. To the inexperienced, it may offer the suggestion needed for him to excise devitalized tissue and skin margins before suturing the wound, particularly a contaminated wound.

Small retractors.
Allis forceps.
Hemostats.
Scissors.
Knife handle and blades. The No. 11 Bard-Parker blade is suggested for skin edges although some surgeons will prefer other types.

The above items in addition to needle holders, toothed forceps, and curved round and skin needles will complete the set, with the addition of fine plain gut for ties, fine silk for sutures, and gauze sponges.

Minor Suture Sets: Where small lacerations needing no more than three or four skin sutures are to be treated, very simple sets of needle holder, tissue forceps, scissors, and curved skin needles will suffice.

Splints

The variety need not be great, but there should be appropriate splints for all extremity fractures.

Thomas splints—adults and children.
Wide unbleached muslin or small towels with safety pins for slings on Thomas splints.
Traction hitches.
Coaptation splints—wood or aluminum; various sizes.
Pneumatic splints—while these have not yet had wide acceptance, they are being improved and show promise, particularly for such fractures as may be splinted with pillows (leg and forearm).
Adjustable cervical spine splints or neck collars.

It is important that all personnel be instructed in the use of all splints. This and the matter of local anesthesia might well be subjects for discussion and demonstration at the emergency conferences mentioned in the chapter dealing with this department as an educational center.

Defibrillator and Cardiac Pacemaker

On some occasions, these will prove invaluable. They are worthless, however, unless personnel trained in their use is present. (See Chapter 16 for discussion.)

All items of emergency department equipment should be of first-class quality. The practice of sending to the emergency department equipment that has been discarded elsewhere is to be condemned. Safety should be one of the primary goals in treating emergency patients, and this cannot be assured with substandard equipment.

EQUIPMENT HAZARDS

One of the principal evidences of immaturity on the part of a physician is the thought that the procurement of technical equipment prepares him to carry out any treatment for which such equipment is designed. Instances of this are myriad. One of the author's friends, a successful and capable general surgeon, tells this story of himself. In the early thirties, when the thorax was gaining in popularity as a field for surgical invasion, he went to Europe and observed thoracic surgery for a few weeks, following which he purchased what he describes as "a suitcase full of chest instruments." He returned to his home and circulated the glad tidings that he was going to do thoracic surgery. He practiced in a city and state where previously little work of this type had been done. He states that the expected referrals did not materialize and that after a reasonable period of time he abandoned the idea, gave his equipment to the hospital, and confined his practice to the parts of the body in which he was trained and experienced.

Another such example was that of a physician combining a

large general practice with surgery. He scheduled the resection of an aortic aneurysm in a hospital where even the surgeons who had had formal training were doing no elective vascular surgery. Fortunately he was dissuaded from his plan without the invocation of authority, but the interesting thing was that among the reasons given to justify the rather ambitious procedure was the fact that he had purchased all the required special instruments.

It has been emphasized in the chapter on plans and planning that the construction of facilities and purchase of equipment beyond the skills of the medical staff are wasteful. Not only that, but they may be dangerous. Progress in the field of medical care has been going on steadily for centuries, but the introduction of techniques requiring equipment that is safe only in the hands of those who have been well schooled in its use has taken place mostly in the middle of this century. Some pieces of equipment used in the treatment of cardiac and respiratory emergencies may be lifesaving, but they may carry with them hazards that must be understood and taken into consideration in their use.

The early history of the development of such things as the pacemaker and defibrillator indicates a knowledge much wider than that usually considered in the field of medical education. The pioneers in this field had to be physicists, as well as physiologists and clinicians. Although the early crude machines have been replaced by cabinets containing nicely calibrated and regulated mechanisms which are sold with an instruction book, making it all sound very simple, they still deal with electric currents that can stop a heart as well as start it. Human skin is a fairly good insulator against electric current, but sometimes it is forgotten that the patient on whom the electric current is being used may have his skin punctured by needles or catheters and through these water may be flowing. Water conducts electricity well and this should be remembered when the patient is hooked up to electrical equipment.

Gechman[3] points out that two major flaws in medical electronic equipment are turning up: (1) faulty components in instrumentation and monitoring devices and (2) wiring systems that do not provide maximum protection for the patient.

Failure of adequate grounding of electric wiring is found in many hospitals. The services of an electrical engineer as consultant or advisor in these matters is recommended. There is further discussion of these problems in Chapter 4, on construction and Chapter 16, on cardiac emergencies.

The defibrillator is both a lifesaving device and a dangerous one. Gechman calls attention to some precautions noted by the Cardiac Arrest Committee at the Columbia-Presbyterian Medical Center. These include proper grounding as well as the use of insulating gloves by the operator when he is applying the electrodes. They also recommend that the defibrillator be tested at regular intervals—not just before use, when delay might be dangerous.

It should be stressed in the techniques that the patient's chest should be thoroughly wiped free of any jelly prior to the application of the paddles, and that the patient's hands should not be in contact with the side rails. Randal[4] quotes the National Academy of Sciences as stating that sick people may be "peculiarly susceptible to electricity because of . . . (their) disease or medication." She also reports that this is seldom taken into account by appliance manufacturers who design for the workshop or the home rather than the hospital. The FDA has on record more than 10,000 injuries from medical devices since 1963.

Stanley[5] emphasizes that the hazards of electric currents passing through various portions of the human body may be extreme. He notes under the heading "Microcurrent Shock" that "there is growing evidence that the subtle effects of very small currents are causing an increasing number of deaths." He enumerates the pieces of equipment that may be dangerous as well as the type of wiring. In a second paper,[5] Stanley explains in detail the designing of a safe electrical wiring system for hospitals and elaborates on safety in equipment design. He gives sound advice on the use of a knowledgeable engineer, not only in wiring but in purchasing equipment. Crampton, in Chapter 16, stresses the value of the services of an electrical or biomedical engineer for the protection of both the patient and those caring for him.

Positive-pressure resuscitators, which have been discussed earlier in this chapter, are not as dangerous as the electrical devices we have been discussing. However, they must be used with discretion. It is a good precaution to have an anesthesiologist and cardiologist give careful instruction to those who are to use all these devices. Some have expressed the opinion that such equipment should only be used in "large hospitals." This, of course, is nonsense. The size of the hospital does not determine the skill of the staff. Many large hospitals are more lax in allowing medical and surgical privileges to the untrained than some small hospitals.

Careful as hospitals may be in granting privileges only within the limits of training and experience in the care of inpatients, it is easy to forget this in the emergency department. Here, staff members of limited training are more likely to be working without supervision than they would be in the operating room or on the wards. Furthermore, some patients arriving in the emergency department are less able to withstand the stresses and strains of treatment than those who have been prepared beforehand and have come to the hospital for scheduled procedures. Their unscheduled appearance does not lessen their right to have the benefit of the most capable and safest treatment that can be provided. It is to be hoped that interest will increase in the quality of care in emergency departments and that it will take precedence over the wave of planning to make room for all the people coming there for all kinds of ailments. This increase of interest should embrace not only the supplying of superior equipment but the training of a maximum number of capable individuals in its appropriate and safe use.

A new monthly publication,[6] *Health Devices,* devoted to the impartial evaluation of medical equipment, was introduced in April 1971. This is a nonprofit service of the Emergency Care Research Institute, 913 Walnut Street, Philadelphia. Pa. The new journal is expensive, $250.00 per year, but this fee will underwrite investigation as well as publication. No advertisements will support it, so the projected reports on such things as patient's monitoring systems, chest pumps, operating tables, suction machines, and other equipment should be unbiased.

REFERENCES

1. Hedstrand, U.: Model studies of artificial ventilation in nerve gas victims. *Forsvarsmedicin, 4*:117–123, 1968.
2. Manually operated resuscitators. *Health Devices, 1*:15, 1971.
3. Gechman, R.: The tiny flaws in medical design can kill. *Resp Physiol,* pp. 89–93, 1968.
4. Randal, Judith: Medical gadgets. Devices introduce electrical hazards. *Newark (N.J.) News,* May 8, 1970.
5. Stanley, P.E.: Electrical shock hazards, I and II. *Hospitals, 45*:58–63, 1971.
6. Editorial: Health devices. *J Trauma, 11*:128, 1971.

Chapter 6

SUPPLIES

In the previous chapter, permanent or semipermanent items have been considered. In fiscal planning, these would fall into the category of capital expenditures. This chapter will deal with the material items which are expendable and that come in the category of operating expenses. In budgetary planning for the purpose of determining hospital charges in the emergency department, thought should be given to depreciation and obsolescence of permanent and semipermanent equipment. Supplies which are used up in the daily operation of the department must, of course, be a factor in computing the cost of operation. This factor will be a major determinant in the estimation of hospital charges.

As suggested in Chapter 12 on costs and fees, most hospitals will establish a minimum figure on which the hospital charges for emergency department services are based. In the opinion of the author, some hospitals make a mistake in not including in this basic fee some charge for supplies. It becomes difficult to explain to patients the extras that are added to the basic fee on the itemized bill, if these extras are obviously of little monetary value. Patients may object to an extra charge of $4.00 because an elastic bandage was supplied, and they cannot be blamed. Much better to include in the basic fee enough to cover things of small value. The hospital is not in the retail medical and surgical supply business and if it were, a 400 percent markup is too high. When the "extra" provided is .5 cc of Adrenalin introduced through a twenty-five cent disposable syringe or a tiny amount of some mass-produced vaccine, the supplementary charge should not be $3.00 to $5.00. The argument that this includes the services of a trained nurse who gives the shot is not valid. "Nursing service," along with the other overhead expenses has already been included in the basic charge. It is not fair to charge for the nurse just because she stands there and looks pretty. Any girl-watcher will tell you that this service is free downtown on any corner. The basic fee includes the nurse's service, and giving a shot should surely be absorbed in this. When the whole deal includes a sizeable amount of a nurse's time in assisting the doctor either in diagnostic procedures or treatment, the picture, of course, changes. No time-cost schedule will be suggested here, but each department should establish some kind of guideline to cover this. The point is that it is much easier to defend a basic charge that is sufficient to include a reasonable amount of expendable supplies, than it is to explain an unreasonable figure for "extras." An elastic bandage has an understandable monetary value and may be charged for but within reason. It is the doctor's job to put it on, and this goes in his fee.

In an effort to prevent the expendable supplies from becoming a financial burden to the department, they must be requisitioned intelligently. A capable purchasing department which usually serves the entire hospital is the best source of aid in requisitioning. Quantities should be enough to assure that supplies are always available and yet not such that the emergency department becomes a second central supply room or a warehouse. There should be some kind of a perpetual inventory that keeps those responsible for reordering informed of approaching shortages. Those responsible for ordering should keep informed of advances in technical matters and the availability of improved items of supply. This calls for direct contact with the suppliers. Unless the purchasing agent has an unusual background, he or she will not have the knowledge to decide if a new item is worthy of trial. Only those who use the items have this knowledge and they should make these decisions. Throughout this book the author has tried to stress the point that important decisions should be made by the people who are involved. Their positions or titles are not important. Many infantry corporals know much more about weapons than the commanding general, who may have come into his command through channels that did not include use of the M-1 rifle or the Browning automatic rifle. The author recalls clearly a personal example of this in the military. His unit had a supply officer who had worked up from the rank of sergeant in peacetime to warrant officer in war. He tried to decide what equipment the orthopedists in the unit should use in treating fractures of the femur. We got him straightened out, but it made him unhappy.

In Chapter 5, the equipment was divided into the "big things" and the "smaller things." Disposable supplies may better be classified into "drugs" and "non-drugs." Like the items of equipment, the list of supplies should be determined by those who are to use them, or at least by experienced members of the medical staff who are conversant with their uses. In the selection of pharmaceuticals, the hospital pharmacist, if there is one, will be a valuable advisor.

THE DRUGS

The *Hospital Formulary,* published by the American Society of Hospital Pharmacists, was used by the American Hospital Association in selecting pharmaceuticals to be listed in its emergency department guide.[1] This list, which is arranged under therapeutic subheadings, is reproduced here in its entirety. From it, the emergency department committee or hospital pharmacy committee, by additions and deletions, may easily prepare a functional list suited to the uses of the professional group working in the emergency department. For cogent reasons, certain drugs may be ruled out by action of the Medical Staffs of some hospitals. These are internal decisions subject to local opinion but should be adhered to in making up this list. This is in line with the philosophy advocated elsewhere in this book, that the emergency department patient deserves the same care and precautions that apply elsewhere in the hospital.

The hospital probably has a pharmacy committee. This committee should review decisions made by the emergency department committee to stock any drugs that are not in the *Hospital Formulary* or drug list approved by the medical staff. This keeps the responsibility in proper channels and guards against the use of dangerous or questionable drugs that may have been advocated for use in certain emergency situations, and it is just another attempt to protect the emergency department patient. The working hours of the hospital pharmacy and its proximity to the emergency department will influence the completeness of the stock. The American Hospital Association list is more complete than most departments would require but will serve as a basis from which the drug list may be chosen. It follows:

Antihistaminics

Diphenhydramine hydrochloride
Promethazine hydrochloride N.F.

Autonomic Drugs

Atropine Sulphate
Dihydroergotamine
Ephedrine sulfate
Epinephrine
Levarterenol bitartrate
Neostigmine bromide
Neostigmine methylsulfate
Phenylephrine hydrochloride

Blood Derivatives and Plasma Expanders

Albumin, normal human serum
Dextran
Fibrinogen, human
Plasma, antihemophilic, human
Plasma, protein fraction, human

Blood Coagulation

Anticoagulants:
    Heparin sodium
Antiheparin agents:
    Hexadimethrine bromide

Protamine sulfate
Tolonium chloride
Hemostatics:
Thrombine

Cardiovascular Drugs*

Amyl nitrite
Digitoxin
Digoxin
Glyceryl trinitrate
Procainamide hydrochloride
Quinidine sulfate

Central Nervous System Drugs

Analgesics:
Acetylsalicylic acid
Acetylsalicylic compound (A.P.C.)
Codeine
Meperidine hydrochloride
Morphine sulfate
Anticonvulsants:
Magnesium sulfate
Phenobarbital
Phenobarbital sodium
Narcotic antagonists:
Nalorphine hydrochloride
Psychotherapeutic agents:
Chlorpromazine hydrochloride
Meprobamate
Respiratory and Cerebral Stimulants:
Ammonia, aromatic spirit
Amphetamine sulfate
Caffeine and sodium benzoate
Methamphetamine hydrochloride
Nikethamide
Picrotoxin, N.F.
Sedatives and hypnotics:
Chloral hydrate
Paraldehyde
Thiopental sodium

* See Chapter 16, Table I, for more complete list.

Electrolitic, Caloric and Water Balance

Replacement solutions:
Dextrose
Sodium chloride
Sodium lactate
Water, purified (for solutions)

Enzymes

Hyaluronidase

Expectorants

Terpine hydrate N.F.

Eye, Ear, Nose and Throat Preparations

Antibiotics:
Bacitracin
Neomycin sulfate
Sulfonamides:
Sulfacetamide sodium
Anti-infectives:
Benzalkonium chloride
Silver nitrate
Anti-inflammatory agents:
Cortisone acetate
Hydrocortisone acetate
Local anesthetics:
Cocaine hydrochloride
Phenol
Tetracaine hydrochloride
Mouth washes and gargles:
Hydrogen peroxide solution
Zinc chloride N.F.
Vasoconstrictors:
Ephedrine sulfate N.F.
Epenephrine
Phenephrine hydrochloride
Unclassified agents:
Fluorescein sodium

Gastrointestinal Drugs

Antacids and absorbants:
   Magnesium magma
   Sodium bicarbonate
Antidiarrhea agents:
   Kaolin with pectine mixture N.F.
Cathartics:
   Glycerine (suppositories)
Emetics:
   Apomorphine hydrochloride

Heavy Metal Antagonists

Dimercaprol
Edathamil calcium-disodium

Hormones and Synthetic Substitutes

Calcium gluconate
Insulin
Parathyroid
Prednisolone
Vasopressin

Local Anesthetics

Ethyl chloride (spray)
Lidocaine hydrochloride
Procaine hydrochloride
Tetracaine hydrochloride

Oxytocics

Ergonovine maleate
Oxytocin

Serums, Toxoids and Vaccines

Antivenin, snake bite, polyvalent
Antivenin, spider bite
Gas gangrene antitoxin, pentavalent
Globulin, immune serum

Tetanus antitoxin, bovine
Tetanus antitoxin, equine
Tetanus toxoid

Skin and Mucous Membrane Preparations

Antibiotic preparations
Benzalkonium chloride
Benzoin
Calamine
Collodion
Dusting powder, absorbable
Film, absorbable gelatin
Hexachlorophene
Iodochlorhydroxyquin
Iodine
Isopropyl alcohol
Methylrosanaline chloride
Nitrofurazone N.F.
Nystatin
Peruvian balsam
Potassium permanganate
Prednisolone
Salicylic acid
Silver nitrate
Silver protein N.F.
Soap, medicinal soft
Talc
Titanium dioxide

Spasmolytics

Papaverine hydrochloride

Vitamins

Phytonadione

THE NON-DRUGS

Among the expendable items outside the pharmaceutical
field surgical dressings comprise the largest group, although
sutures, soaps, detergents, and other things are included.
Surgical dressings have undergone remarkable changes in

the past two decades. These changes involve both quality and variety. There was a time when adhesive tape was thick, tough, and often irritant to some skins. Now it may be obtained in forms that are thin, porous, seldom irritating, and very easy to apply. The form in which it is supplied has also been greatly improved. Time was when the nurse or doctor reached over to a shelf and probably picked up a three to four-inch five-yard roll and tore off the length wanted. If a narrower width was desired, they may have ripped the piece lengthwise. Now the far superior tape is supplied in widths from one-half to four inches, in wall dispensing holders that make it easy to cut lengths exactly to fit the need. These are refillable, so the dispensers need not be discarded when they are empty. It is poor economy to use loose rolls of adhesive. Employee time is the big element in hospital costs today, so anything that cuts this down is economical. The several manufacturers supply adhesive tape with varying features, but it is all good. A careful study of the dispensers is as important as selection of the type of tape.

Bandages have not changed so much as adhesive tape over the years, but here again the method of supply has changed. There is no use in buying the neatly packaged bandages of different widths such as one would want in a first aid kit where they might not be used for considerable periods of time. They may be bought more economically in yard-wide rolls wrapped in paper and cut to various widths. These may be broken up into the various sizes and kept in bins or boxes for convenient use. We are referring here to ordinary gauze bandages. Another bandage that has gained great popularity since World War II is the slightly elastic gauze bandage known in the trade as "kling." These make a neater cover for dressed wounds and are more comfortable because of their ability to conform to the surface. While they do not remain in place without a piece of adhesive, they do cling, as the name suggests, and will not slide as ordinary gauze may when placed on an arm or leg that tapers. They are well worth the slight extra cost for many dressings. Other bandages that should be supplied in any emergency department are flannel, muslin, and elastic adhesive bandages. They all have their specific purposes and fit well-defined needs. Along with bandages, we may include stockinette of various sizes and weights. There is a type of stockinette ("tube gauze") much lighter than that used under plaster casts that is most convenient for certain dressings, particularly on hands and feet, as well as for retaining scalp dressings. These may also be obtained in wall dispensers that hold different widths and make cutting to size an easy task.

Plaster-of-paris bandages are, of course, used daily in emergency departments and should be available in the fracture room. Those of us who did fracture work in the twenties and early thirties can remember when these were made by rolling gauze bandages through powdered plaster of paris and then storing them in a dry place. This activity has gone the same way as the folding of gauze, the sharpening of hypodermic needles, and other time-consuming procedures indulged in by hospital personnel in the days of low pay scales. The last time I saw plaster dressings being made by hand was in Truetta's clinic in the Radcliffe Infirmary in Oxford, England, in 1943. Even then, these were really not bandages, but specially shaped plaster slabs for shoulder spicas, and other irregularly shaped plaster dressings. Few nurses or other people would have the patience and the ability to make these today. In the last fifteen or twenty years, substitutes for plaster-of-paris bandages have been put on the market and have gained some popularity because of their lack of weight. These are made from various materials, some quick-drying and some not. Decision as to whether these should be stocked will be made by the surgeons who would use them, but they are all expensive as compared to good plaster bandages.

Gauze dressings for all types and sizes of wounds are now available in individual sterile packages or in packages containing several dressings. Both single and multiple packages may well be obtained and used as the situation demands. They probably cost no more than gauze purchased in bulk and sterilized in metal jars and their sterility is more dependable. These would not be practical in a major operating room where they are used in much greater numbers and where sponge counts are routine, but for emergency department dressings they have replaced the bulk gauze sponges in many hospitals. The old method of cutting a 4 × 4 gauze pad to size for smaller dressings is passé. Smaller pads are available and are time savers and much neater. Several makes of small- to medium-sized dressings in circular, square, and rectangular shapes and adherent to adhesive strips are available in sterile form. These are not only time savers but are neat and comfortable. Patients appreciate them, as they usually result in a smaller dressing than one put together with gauze and separate adhesive. This is all part of the good impression that should be made on these one-trip patients, who will probably not be seen again. These items are also supplied in convenient wall dispensers, one of which is shown on the wall at the Radcliffe Infirmary in Figure 22. It may seem that a large variety of wall-attached dressing dispensers is being advocated, but it must be remembered that if they are not provided, all of these various dressings will have to be tucked away in drawers or strewn along shelves where they may not always be just where they are wanted. Emergency department medicine is usually not a leisurely activity. Anything that will help the doctors and nurses to finish treatment of one patient and get on to the next is good planning.

The subject of surgical dressings should not be dropped without mention of a large gauze dressing that is most useful for covering areas on the abdomen, thorax, or thigh. This is a sterile dressing and has its most important use in covering large burned areas. It may be used in its full dimensions or may be folded if the area is smaller. Many ambulance crews have found this dressing convenient and time saving where otherwise they would have had to apply a number of smaller-sized dressings to a large area.

Unless the department is a new one in a new hospital, with a newly organized or recruited staff, the personnel will know from experience what dressings and other supplies have proven most useful. While no plea is made for purchasing everything the suppliers offer, it is suggested that the variety be such as to provide convenient, easily applied, and comfortable dressings for all types of wounds. The matter of comfort is not a minor one.

The selection of surgical sutures will require some thought and planning. If much emergency department work is to be done by plastic surgeons, they may want types of sutures not required by others, with emphasis on small sizes. The wishes of all physicians should, within reason, be recognized in selecting sutures. After all, the neatness of the healed wounds is the doctor's trademark, and he has a right to make this as good as possible. The only warning that comes to mind in this connection is to weigh carefully what may seem to be unreasonable demands from young surgeons fresh out of training. Occasionally they have left the mother house with fixed opinions that if wounds are not treated just as they were at the university, the results will be disastrous. Give them some of what they want, but if their demands are ridiculous, there is no better time than the present to start shaping these young men. Some of them will make good doctors when they learn that there are two ways to do most things.

Adequate amounts of the various supplies should be kept in the supply room, if the department is large enough to have such a room. However, as stated in Chapter 3, this is no substitute for "well stocked cabinets within easy reach of the patients' stretchers." This is where the action is, and this is where the supplies are needed. This goes for all rooms, large or small and regardless of their labels. Just because a room is planned for care of cardiac or fracture cases does not guarantee that patients treated there may not need surgical dressings. The possibility of a variety of injuries is the reason flexibility has been stressed in the planning of all treatment rooms or areas.

Some of the items listed under "The Smaller Things" in Chapter 5 on equipment might have been included here as expendable supplies. However, the following list is made up of things not listed in Chapter 5 and that will require frequent replacement.

Dressings

Adhesive tape, assorted widths.
Adhesive, moleskin.
Adhesive elastic bandages—2, 3, and 4-inch

Adhesive solvent.
Bandages, elastic—2 to 6-inch.
Bandages, flannel.
Bandages, gauze—1 to 4-inch.
Bandages, Kling—1 to 6-inch.
Bandages, muslin—3, 4, and 6-inch.
Bandages, plaster—2 to 6-inch.
Bandages, triangular.
Band-Aids—assorted sizes and shapes.
Cotton and cotton balls.
Eye patches and protectors.
Felt, orthopedic.
Gauze, packing.
Gauze, vaseline.
Splints, plaster—3 x 15 to 5 x 45 inches.
Sponges (dressings)—assorted sizes.
Sponges (nonadherent), Telfa—assorted sizes.
Stockinette, 2 to 10 inches.
Tube gauze—assorted widths.

Glassware

Connectors, glass or plastic.
Droppers, medicine.
Thermometers, oral and rectal.
Slides, microscopic.
Test tubes—sterile (for cultures).
Urine specimen bottles.

Rubber Goods

Catheters, assorted sizes.
Catheters, Foley, assorted sizes.
Finger cots.
Heels, rubber—for walking casts.
Tips for crutches.
Tubing, intravenous.
Tubing for stethoscopes.

Miscellaneous

Applicators, cotton-tipped.
Armboards.
Belts, rib—assorted sizes.

Brushes, hand.
Canes.
Crutches.
Cups, paper.
Depressors, tongue.
Enemas, Fleet.
Ether (for solvent).
Gloves, rubber and plastic.
Jelly, lubricating.
pHisoHex.
Powder, Biosorb.
Pins, safety.
Slings.
Towels.

Sutures

Chromic gut—assorted sizes.
Plain gut—assorted sizes.
Nylon—assorted sizes.
Silk—assorted sizes.

REFERENCE

1. *The Emergency Department in the Hospital: A Guide to Organization and Management.* Chicago, American Hospital Association, 1962.

Chapter 7

STAFFING THE EMERGENCY DEPARTMENT

Important as the construction, physical equipment, and supplies of this department are, it is the staffing that is of greatest importance in determining its effectiveness. Staffing includes not only physicians, but nurses, technicians and others.

DOCTORS

Since the department, as well as the hospital as a whole, cannot function without doctors, and since they present the biggest problem, they will be considered first. There are two facets of the physician coverage of an emergency department that must be considered separately as well as in relationship to each other, the economic and the quality of patient care.

The Economic Facet

Shall patients other than the medically indigent pay for professional care (that is, aside from the charge for hospital service)?

If so, how much, and who shall set the fees?

How shall these fees be collected?

If the patients do not pay separately for professional services, shall the hospital charge be increased so that they do not get too great a bargain?

Who shall determine which patients cannot pay, that is, who are medically indigent?

If patients are not charged a professional fee, are the doctors expected to render this service gratis?

These are only some of the economic considerations that will come up. No attempt will be made to give a dogmatic answer to any of them or even to suggest an answer to all of them. The problem as a whole will be discussed with the hope that this will guide the thinking of administrators and emergency room committees. Let it first be noted that the doctors are to provide this service, something that no one else can provide, so they should have a large voice in the fee planning. On the other hand, it would seem reasonable that they should be willing to allow several factors to influence their decisions.

There are two viewpoints from which the hospital-physician relationship may be considered. One of these viewpoints taken by many administrators and trustees leads them to feel that doctors should be so grateful for the hospital facilities provided that they should be willing to pay for them. This is evidenced by mandatory assessments made on doctors in some hospital fund drives. Fortunately, this is not a widespread custom, and in many cases it has not improved staff-trustee relationships. Although demanding money payments from doctors may seem high-handed, it does not seem out of line to expect them to contribute certain services in the hospital. Physicians are usually willing to do this with respect to the medically indigent either as inpatients or outpatients. It is when a plan of free service for all comers in the emergency department is proposed that some physicians will balk.

The second viewpoint from which the hospital-physician relationship may be seen is the one from which it is clear that without doctors a hospital is not a hospital. Some people go to a hospital without realizing this, yet it will not be long before they ask for a doctor if one does not present himself. Any other group may be removed and, although this will hinder patient care and will inconvenience the doctors, the doctors can still take care of sick people. They know their indispensability, yet it is to be hoped that they seldom have to flaunt it. Fortunate is the hospital where staff, administrator, and trustees are willing to subordinate their personal interests to the extent that a spirit of friendly cooperation prevails. The most important party in the whole maneuver, the patient, will profit. It is the patient for whom the hospital exists.

The author makes no apology for the above philosophical

discussion. It is presented solely as a means of aiding emergency department planners to appoach this problem of staffing with open minds. As in the planning of the physical facilities, it will help to come to an agreement regarding the purpose of the emergency department beyond the actual care of patients. Is it to be fitted into the whole hospital program as a feature of public relations? Is it to be operated as a loss leader, so to speak? New hospitals may be tempted to take this attitude. The writer remembers a fine hospital that opened its doors in New York State several decades ago. The community had not previously had a first-class hospital, and not only the public but the profession needed to be educated with regard to the value of certain hospital services. The trustees voted to give patients, even pay-ward patients, all the x-ray and laboratory services that their doctors might order, if they stayed a week or longer. Ward beds were $4.00 per day, so a patient might come in and, by paying as little as $28.00, receive a week's board and room with excellent nursing care and laboratory and x-ray services that today would run well into three figures. This bargain was discontinued after a limited period of time.

It is not likely that many hospitals today will plan to operate the emergency department without at least breaking even. It is likely that if the department does not pay for itself, a study will be made leading to a change in policy. It is obvious, however, that the economy of an emergency department includes both hospital and professional services and that a clear-cut policy must be established with regard to both. Fees and charges will be discussed in another chapter. The subject has been introduced here as it must be considered in planning the professional staff.

Patient Care: Its Quality

This second facet of professional care is not mentioned last because it is of lesser importance. On the contrary, all conscientious individuals, whether personally involved or not, will give quality of patient care the highest priority.

Many methods of staffing emergency departments have

proved successful, but not in all instances. Some of these are
the following:

1. Intern and resident coverage.
2. "Moonlighting residents."
3. A rotating roster of the active staff on a fee-for-service
basis or at fixed salary rates.
4. A volunteer roster from the staff.
5. A contract or concession with a small group of doctors—
working only in the emergency department.
6. Staff physicians on salary to cover the emergency department, with salaries paid by the hospital but with patients
billed in the name of the doctors and the fees going to the
hospital.

Intern and Resident Coverage

Where the hospital has a well-supervised program of intern
and resident training, this may be quite successful. Several
features should, however, be included in such a plan. Emergency room responsibility should not be placed on the shoulders of first-year interns without strict supervision by experienced
residents or members of the attending staff. Whereas in much
of his work with inpatients the intern has time to go to the
library or otherwise seek assistance, he will have to act on the
spot in the emergency department. This is not to say that he
should not serve a period of time here. He may, but under certain restrictions that will protect the patient, particularly from
errors of omission. Even a resident, who may be in the third
year of his training, should have certain checks to prevent his
overenthusiasm or lack of experience from leading him astray.
These checks or restrictions should be put down in writing in
emergency department rules. They should apply particularly
to the handling of complicated fractures as well as injuries to
other than the skeletal system that might produce disabilities.
The arrangements for adequate consultation and assistance
from the attending staff should be definite. Responsibilities
should be assigned to certain designated staff members for definite periods.

Unless the hospital is in a community where it is serving

largely medically indigent patients, the matter of fees for professional services must be thought of with resident-staff coverage. These men are frequently not licensed, and while it is legal for them to care for patients with the hospital taking the responsibility, it may be illegal to make a charge for their services. It would be a good policy to have the opinion of the hospital counsel on this matter. When the attending-staff member comes in and participates in the care, either by directing the resident, assisting him, or doing the treatment himself, he is surely rendering a service worthy of a fee, if the plan allows charges to private patients. The author does not believe that a charge is in order if he only gives advice to the resident over the telephone, although he has heard this practice defended. Policies should be adopted in all of these situations to free the hospital from liability or even criticism and to standardize the procedures.

As will be mentioned in the chapter on the emergency department as an educational center, interns and residents may profit greatly from experience received here, but one of the biggest problems to be considered is how much responsibility they should assume and how their services should be rated in the charge column. The widespread insurance coverage now found among people who were once considered "clinic-type patients" has changed the thinking of some of these people. They know that funds are available to cover their emergency room care. Some of them will demand the best. If we still believe in the time-honored patient-physician relationship and free choice of physician, we will try to see that they get it.

A discussion of resident coverage of emergency departments is not complete without reference to the foreign resident. The entrance of the foreign-born and educated young doctor into the American medical scene since World War II has presented several problems. An injustice is done to some of these intelligent and industrious young men and women in implying that they are inferior in ability to American-born and educated interns. If the tables were turned and some of us were thrust into emergency departments in foreign hospitals, we would be at a disadvantage. It must be granted, however, that where they have language difficulties, foreign residents are particularly handicapped in the emergency department. They may not be able to get an accurate history, although this is more important to them than it is to the police and the press. The author[1] has emphasized elsewhere that the history may play a definite part in the diagnosis and treatment of injured patients. To witness the efforts of a young doctor, not well versed in the English language, trying to find out how someone got hurt may be amusing, but it is also sobering. The information sought may be the key to a correct diagnosis. This situation is further proof that supervision in the emergency department is essential to good patient care.

"Moonlighting" Residents

Some hospitals lacking a resident staff and unable to work out a satisfactory plan of attending-staff coverage have resorted to use of residents from elsewhere. This plan, while having a number of drawbacks, has proven workable in some places. Residents from nearby hospitals are engaged at set fees for fixed hours of service during their time off. These are usually the night hours, and the "moonlighting" residents work on their nights off. The chief of surgery in one community hospital on the fringe of a metropolitan area explained to the author that his hospital had an approved intern program but no residency program. Some of their former interns take residencies in teaching hospitals in the city and welcome the opportunity to come back and take the eight-hour night shift in the emergency department for $50.00. They are at home in the hospital where they interned and thus do not require a period of indoctrination to adapt themselves to work there. The hospital gets doctors of known ability, and the residents get experience as well as an addition to their incomes. This plan will not be possible in 1975, when internships without residencies will no longer be approved.

While this unique system has some good features, there are some strong arguments on the debit side. Many residents need the night off from responsibility for rest and recreation. The wives and children of married residents profit from the extra dollars, but they lose the normal companionship that comes with family life. The resident years are a strain on all concerned in these families and, while one facet of this is the limited financial resources, another is the all too frequent absence of the young husband and father from the family circle. The latter is compounded when the resident adds to his working hours. The cost of a medical education plus the sacrifices attendant upon prolonged specialty training have created obstacles that seem insurmountable to many talented young men and women today. It is small wonder that some of them feel impelled to seek extra income from any available sources; yet it is to be hoped that not many will have to seek this through adding to an already burdensome program of work. The professional coverage of emergency departments by "moonlighting" residents is not the ideal solution.

A Rotating Roster

Since only one in five hospitals in this country has interns or residents, the responsibility for professional coverage usually falls on the attending staff. Some plan for spreading this responsibility must be adopted to prevent it from becoming too much of a burden on anyone. A rotating roster of staff physicians is the most popular system. The economic aspects of this system will be discussed in another chapter, but the staff must agree on this so there is some uniformity of charges.

The universal acceptance of rotation of all M.D.'s by all of the active staff members would make this arrangement easy to put into effect, but two questions arise that are of major importance. First, in order to lessen the frequency with which staff members have to serve, shall all members of the staff be required to take their turns? Second, are all members of the staff (regardless of their specialties) capable of rendering the type and quality of professional service desired and expected?

Some doctors will insist that everyone including the anesthesiologist, radiologist, pathologist, and ophthalmologist should participate. The answer to the second question may provide the answer to the first. Nothing said here should be interpreted as a reflection on the four specialists mentioned or on any representatives from these specialists on general hospital staffs, when it comes to activities in their specialties. Perhaps I have used these specialists as examples because I have had the responsibility of deciding on their assignment in making out emergency department rosters. I have had staff members—particularly senior members beginning to feel their age—demand that all M.D.'s serve, and I have had the interesting experience of having a representative of one of these specialties refuse to take his turn on the excuse that it would interfere with his appointments! The fact that the surgeons and internists had appointments did not seem to have occurred to him. It was interesting because this particular staff member had often complained that he was not recognized as a doctor but only as a technician. It would seem that serving on the emergency roster would have given him the status that he wished, particularly if he had to get up at night, a practice in which he lacked recent experience. In the interests of prospective patients, he was allowed to retain his status as a "technician," although some of the staff were not happy about the decision.

There are some doctors who always retain an interest in the whole patient and to a certain extent keep abreast of what is going on outside their own specialties. Others assume the attitude fitting the definition that a specialist is a doctor who claims to know nothing about medicine outside his own specialty. Can these men, who may for years have limited their professional activities to a narrow channel, be expected to render adequate care to the broad spectrum of cases coming to the emergency department? Certainly the anesthesiologist should be able to recognize and treat shock in the badly injured patient. He would also know by observation what surgeons do in many of these situations, but could he reduce a Colles' fracture, suture extensor tendons (leaving flexor tendons for the surgeon in the operating room), and do an emergency tube thoracostomy to alleviate asphyxia from pneumothorax? The radiologist could surely diagnose a trimalleolar fracture of the ankle and tell when it was properly reduced, but could be mold the fragments into place and apply the cast? Could he insert a

Kirchner wire and pull down the lower half of a fractured femur? The pathologist, if he were the clinical variety and not just a tissue pathologist, might be just the man to diagnose an obscure case of poisoning, particularly if he had worked as a medical examiner, but such cases are rare compared to burns, fractures, and lacerations. He would be experienced in describing a ruptured hollow viscus at autopsy, but it might have been a long time since he had seen one of these victims alive. Could the ophthalmologist be expected to distinguish between a bruise of the left flank and a possible ruptured spleen? These questions practically answer themselves and point to the conclusion that unless these men were exceedingly conscientious about calling for help, they might not render the desired quality of care even if they were willing to get up at night. It might be better to have them do their bit as consultants in their specialties and to retain the general practitioners, surgeons, and internists as front-line troops.

So it seems reasonable to agree that where an adequate number of physicians of broader experience are available, they had better make up the emergency department roster. To be sure the quality of care will fluctuate among surgeons and the others assigned to these tasks, but an attempt should be made to keep it on a high level. In large hospitals, completely departmentalized, it may be possible to have rosters in various specialties on call, but an M.D. must see the patient and decide whom to call unless the decision is so obvious that it may be made by the nurse in charge.

A Volunteer Roster

Troubles in getting equal cooperation in this department from the entire staff have led some hospitals to organize a group of volunteers from the staff. It may be expected that all of these will cooperate, otherwise they would not have volunteered. Abbott[2] has reported the success of this method at the Pontiac (Michigan) General Hospital. In this 381-bed hospital, a call for volunteers resulted in the formation of an association known as the Professional Medical Service Group made up of about 25 staff doctors. This group consisted largely of general practitioners, surgeons, and internists, but other specialties were represented. They were mostly young men, and all had had emergency department experience during their intern or resident training. Being young and not yet completely busy with their private practices, they had time for this work, and it augmented their incomes. The professional fees collected for them by an accounting firm were pooled, and the doctors were paid fixed hourly fees for the time they were on duty. Abbott pointed out that by the time the patient had paid the minimum charge of $6.00 to the hospital and the minimum professional fee of $4.00, he was getting less for his money than if he had gone to a doctor's office, but that this had not seemed to reduce the traffic to the emergency department.

Abbott's first report was made soon after the plan was activated. He[3] has more recently reported their five-year experience. The basic plan has changed little, although the fees have gone up. Five obstetricians and gynecologists have now joined the group as have three pediatricians. Their average age is 36. The group has incorporated and has adopted a constitution and bylaws as well as a set of rules and regulations. The group meets quarterly and the Board of Directors more frequently. Hospital management meets at intervals with the board to discuss the quality of patient care. An accounting firm still does the billing for the group, using the Michigan Blue Shield schedule as a guide. The members of the group receive $16.00 per hour for their services while on duty. Originally they had received $10.00. There is now a waiting list of doctors wanting to participate.

The incorporated group carries malpractice insurance. Abbott reports that the plan has resulted in a high quality of patient care around the clock. The administrator feels that they have the best professional coverage of the emergency department in the 55 years that the hospital has served the community. This plan has been copied in many places.

Wesson[4] reports a similar method to be successful at the Mountainside Hospital, Montclair, New Jersey. A volunteer panel of sixteen physicians provides emergency room care. They were paid $10.00 per hour at the time of reporting several years ago for the eight-hour shifts which they serve. The service is administered by the Department of General Practice. The panel members observe the call system for specialties in vogue in the hospital. When interns are assigned to the emergency department, the staff members use the emergency department patients as a means of teaching traumatology and emergency room care. Each patient is given the opportunity to have his private physician if he prefers. If the patient requires admission to the hospital and does not have a private doctor, the emergency room doctor may admit him as his own patient, if he is qualified to care for the particular condition. This plan, which has the enthusiastic support of the entire staff, was adopted after study of many plans over the country.

A Contract or Concession with a Small Group of Doctors

Ingenious new plans are usually the result of failures of more common ones. A plan that now seems to be a happy solution to this problem in many places is that of granting an emergency department concession to a small group of doctors who will give full time to this activity. A contract or other binding agreement is made between this group and the hospital. The doctors do not have offices outside the hospital and have no inpatient privileges. Neither do they make house calls. In other words, they become emergency room specialists and devote full time to their specialty. A group of four doctors can work out an eight-hour shift (in some places it is 12 hours) schedule under this arrangement, with no one having to work too long hours and with little difficulty in arranging weekend and vacation time off. Rules must be adopted and followed about patients who come to the emergency room and ask for physicians not in the group. There should also be fixed rules about calling for consultants or other help where the services required appear to be beyond the experience and skill of the doctor on duty. These are details that may be worked out in the same way that staff rules are adopted. To the surprise of some, this plan has furnished very satisfactory incomes to the physicians involved and has produced good service. Needless to say, as time goes on, the group doctors become more skilled in caring for the kinds of cases they see in this department. With this arrangement, direct billing by the doctors involved is usually followed, although the hospital may do this for them on the doctors' billheads. The doctors' services stop with the first treatment. Patients, unless they are admitted, are then referred to physicians of their own choice.

The Alexandria (Virginia) Hospital was the first to report success with this plan. Mills[5] reports that this 288-bed hospital is in a community of 100,000 population. Because the medical-staff rotation plan had not been successful, four members of the staff engaged in private practice agreed to assume responsibility for emergency room care. The following rules were agreed upon by the staff and the contracting physicians:

1. Emergency department physicians will see every patient who presents himself, except that

    A. Patients having private physicians will be treated only at the request of the patient's doctor. (The nursing staff makes a telephone search for the doctor.)

    B. No continuing course of therapy will be undertaken.

2. Emergency physicians have the *right** and *obligation** to call on consultants of the staff when this is in the patients' best interests.

3. These arrangements will in no way alter the traditional right of staff members to treat their own patients in the emergency department.

4. The emergency department physicians will not engage in private practice except within the department.

The emergency department physicians at Alexandria make charges "in keeping with those of the area and with the Blue Shield schedule." These and the hospital charges are presented separately to the patient, and Mills reports that the dual charge acts as a deterrent to excessive use of the facility or the use of the service in preference to a doctor's office. This is in contrast to Abbott's report from Pontiac. Indigent patients are not billed, but are paid for by a municipal appropriation. After two years' experience, everyone concerned seemed to be pleased with the arrangement at Alexandria.

    * Author's italics.

Beaven[6] also strongly supports the plan of turning the professional care in the emergency department over to a small group of full-time doctors. His hospital, like the one in Alexandria, is in the densely populated area surrounding the nation's capitol. While this system is spreading in popularity, there is little doubt that in many places its contemplation would bring loud protests. Porter[7] takes a strong stand against the encroachment into private practice by emergency departments. He objects, quite rightly, to the exploitation of private practitioners, by requiring them to care for nonemergency patients who are well able to pay for medical care. Few will take issue with him in his contention that they should not give free care to nonindigent patients, particularly those not having emergencies. His stand would be firmer, however, if he insisted that the doctors make themselves more available, particularly in off-hours, so that patients would not have a valid reason for going to the emergency department for all ailments.

Salaried Staff Physicians

Another method successfully adopted in some hospitals is that of having the hospital pay fixed salaries to physicians who agree to cover the emergency department. To escape the charge of corporate practice of medicine, some arrangement such as billing the patient in the name of the doctor must be made. Objections of organized medicine to hospitals engaging in the corporate practice of medicine have been based on sound reasoning for the most part. In fact, the practice is illegal in some states. The profession has been willing to overlook mild examples of this but has reacted violently against hospitals selling the services of doctors at a profit and thus exploiting their abilities. Of course, no doctor has to be so victimized and, in many instances, medical societies and staffs might well reprimand the doctors who enter into such agreements, rather than the institutions. This is not the place to present the pros and cons of this situation or to take sides in it. Attention is called to the matter as a suggestion that disputes and internal wrangling may be avoided by making sure that the medical staff approves the arrangement. Many of the attending staff may be so happy about escaping what they consider a chore that they will be quite liberal in their judgments concerning the propriety of the arrangements. It is interesting to note how often convenience may influence conscience.

A modified type of the above plan may be to have the salaried doctors cover the night shift while the balance of the staff rotates in the daytime. Just as when the whole staff rotates on call, Plans 4, 5, and 6 should be set up with the clear understanding that the doctors furnishing the professional coverage be limited to such activities as their training and experience warrants. The necessary consultants should be called when needed. The right of a patient to call for the doctor of his choice should also be considered in the rules established, although how much of this right he sacrifices by not trying to contact a physician and coming directly to the hospital for nonemergency conditions is a question worthy of consideration. Allowing patients to come to the hospital at all hours for nonemergency treatments and then allowing them to dictate who shall treat them is surely a surrender of the rights of the hospital and its staff.

Much as I deplore it, I recognize that changes may come in the foreseeable future in the relationship of patients, physicians, and hospitals that may alter any plan adopted. Perhaps there are those who can predict these things. If so, they may be able to offer sound advice to committees planning emergency department coverage. Readers are commended to their advice but warned to weigh it carefully.

As stated at the beginning of this chapter, staffing is the most important facet of emergency department planning. The several months of recruiting and assigning doctors to this most sensitive area in the entire hospital program do not solve the problem just because one of the methods is agreed upon. Getting doctors to agree to serve does not guarantee that their services will be satisfactory. They must not be selected without careful assessment of their capabilities. After they are selected, they must have a full measure of guidance and support.

Opinions differ as to what kind of doctor is best in this assignment. Some think the internist, some the general surgeon, some the pediatrician, although serious as the pediatric problems may be, they are usually much in the minority. There are good arguments in favor of an experienced general practitioner, particularly one who has had some meaningful experience in the field of trauma. As time goes on and this type of practice gains in status, as it surely will, more young doctors will train specifically for it. Until the completely trained emergency doctor becomes available, all those filling the position must have guidelines to follow. Chapter 20 describes a manual of policies and procedures. Such a manual, prepared by physicians in various specialties, will prove invaluable to those using it. It will also serve to protect the physician from criticism. If he follows the directions laid down for him, he will have the support of other members of the medical staff who have written the manual. New appointees to the department must know that unless they have adequate professional reasons to do so, they should not stray very far from the rule book. As they become accustomed to the work in the department and gain the confidence of the specialists in various lines, they will, of course, be able to exert more independence in their directions. There is seldom an exact way that any condition should be treated. We are discussing general principles here. Periodic instructional conferences, with various specialists on the staff leading the discussions, will be of value.

The support that the emergency department doctors require must come from the other members of the medical staff. Being posted on the "On Call" roster is not taken seriously enough by some staff members. It is considered a nuisance by some. This attitude is wrong and should be the subject of administrative investigation, starting with the director of the department. The on-call doctors should even pattern their private practices so as to be available during their periods of duty. It is not good planning to have a surgeon who is "on service" for a given period of time also assigned to the "on call" roster in the emergency department. He may be caring for his service duties when he is badly needed in the emergency department. In one Montana city with two medium-sized hospitals, the author found that the same surgeon was assigned to emergency department duty in both hospitals at the same time. The hospitals did not have full-time doctors in these departments, so the coverage was obviously quite faulty. In another Montana city, I found that they called "whomever they could get" when a patient came into the emergency department. This is poor planning. Good staffing calls for having a doctor on the spot or available within a reasonable time. It also calls for prompt specialty backup when needed, if such specialists are available in the community.

A subcommittee of the National Research Council, on which the author has served, has worked on plans to "categorize" emergency services in areas or communities. This plan is also under consideration by the American Medical Association and the American College of Surgeons. If it reaches the point of wide acceptance and implementation, hospitals—particularly their emergency departments—will be classified with regard to their capabilities in caring for medical and surgical emergencies. Institutions will be placed in Category 1 only if they have the capability of promptly caring for all types of emergencies without reference to assistance from elsewhere. Categories 2, 3, and 4 will have lesser capabilities. The hope is that ambulance crews, police and fire departments, and for that matter the general public will be able to select the institutions to which patients in emergency situations should be taken for complete emergency care and necessary follow-up care after the emergency is dealt with. This will require judgment beyond the capability of many of those who transport the patients, but the plan is a good one if it will work. One danger might be that patients needing immediate lifesaving care might be taken past institutions that could provide that service in order that, after the emergency is over, they could continue their treatment without transfer. In classifying institutions, the availability of a competent staff is recognized as the most important feature in rating one place higher than another.

NURSES

Nurses, like doctors, have likes and dislikes and where possible these should be taken into consideration in assigning them to various departments. Of course, their abilities are to be considered first, but other things being equal, they will work best where they are most contented. Assignment to the emergency department would be most disappointing to some, while to others it would offer a challenge to serve a type of patient in which they had maximum interest.

If an emergency department is devoting most of its effort to the care of true emergencies, the majority of the patients will be surgical and require some type of surgical treatment. The type of nurse who is most capable in the operating room and contented there will likely be happy and capable in the emergency department, but there is one definite difference between the two. Most operations in the regular surgical suite are scheduled in advance and allow time for orderly preparations. Surgical procedures in the emergency department are not only unscheduled but unpredictable. In the course of a few minutes, an emergency department may change from a quiet area, where one or more people are folding gauze, putting away supplies, completing records, or following some other nonexciting pursuit, to a bustling department, with several injured people all needing prompt attention, as well as friends, relatives, ambulance attendants, police, and others milling about. The closest parallel would be the shock and operating tents in a field or evacuation hospital on active duty in wartime. The nurse to whom uncertainty, adventure, and hurried activity offer a challenge is a good choice for this assignment. It is not an assignment for the inexperienced or fainthearted. Student nurses will profit by work here but only under the watchful supervision of seasoned graduates. Particularly for night shifts should the nursing personnel be dependable and experienced. Even though some nights may be slack, there is no way to tell when great responsibilities may have to be assumed. Except in the smallest and most inactive hospitals, the nursing assignments should not be on an on-call basis. The nurse or nurses should be present in person and should have relief at mealtime or when they otherwise have to be temporarily absent.

Nurses who show an aptitude for work of this type may be trained on the job to increase their skills. Not only nursing supervisors but members of the medical staff should be willing to train them. Too often, training and education in the care of the sick and injured is thought of only as something that can be accomplished in formal courses. The emergency department can be an area of continuing education. This is discussed in more detail in another chapter.

OTHER PERSONNEL

There are others besides doctors and nurses who make up the capable emergency department team. Nurses aides, orderlies, and maids may be assigned here, although only in the larger institutions will they likely be full-time. Considerations of interest and adaptability may well guide even temporary assignments. Male attendants who have been trained in first aid and who enjoy such activity will be more valuable than those who prefer to avoid it. Secretaries and receptionists will free nurses for full-time professional duties.

Laboratory and x-ray technicians who from time to time have duties in this department are concerned primarily with carrying out the procedures of their departments and will neither be selected by nor supervised by emergency department authority. It is well to try to maintain a close and friendly working arrangement with these departments at all times. Only in such things as the handling of fracture patients should emergency department personnel offer admonition to x-ray technicians. In their striving for perfection in the taking of films of fractures, some technicians may attempt to position patients in a way that would be deleterious to their condition. They may even want to remove splints at times. This should not be allowed unless a physician is present to maintain traction or otherwise prevent further damage.

To repeat the thought introduced at the beginning of this chapter, the personnel is the most important factor in the efficiency and effectiveness of the emergency department. It is no place to assign second-raters.

REFERENCES

1. Spencer, J.H.: The importance of the history in the diagnosis and treatment of accidental injuries. *Am J Surg, 93*:503–507, 1957.

2. Abbott, V.C.: How to staff a hospital emergency department. *Bull Am Coll Surgeons, 47:4,* 1962, pp. 137–138, 182.
3. Abbott, V.C.: Emergency room staffing. Five year's experience with the Pontiac plan. *Mod Hosp,* 1966.
4. Wesson, H.R.: Personal communication.
5. Mills, J.D.: A method of staffing a community hospital emergency department. *Va Med Mon, 90:*518–519, 1963.
6. Beaven, W.E.: *Med Ann D C, 34:4,* 1965.
7. Porter, R.: Our enemy: the emergency room. *Med Economics,* 1963.

Chapter 8

ADMINISTRATION

O nce constructed, equipped, and even staffed, an emergency department does not automatically run itself. Critics of the very worthy Hill-Burton program have been right in a statement often made to the effect that many Hill-Burton hospitals have been planned and built with a minimum of thought as to how they will be staffed. A Congressional Committee[1] involved with the original Hill-Burton planning was warned about this but seemed to disregard the warning. A well-meaning local governing board has proudly seen the last piece of equipment unpacked and put into position and has turned to the doctors with the remark, "Well, there is your hospital. Now make use of it." It is that board's continuing responsibility both morally and legally to assure that the quality of the work in the hospital matches the quality of the shiny new equipment.

A similar responsibility lies on the shoulders of the committee that plans an emergency department, either to keep an "eagle eye" on its operation or assure that an equally responsible group does this. The committee that assumes the role of advisor to the department when it begins to function may not be the same one mentioned in Chapter 3, which was the planning committee. It may be a new committee or a partially new one. Representatives from medical staff, nursing service, and administration are still appropriate, but the member from the governing board may be dispensed with. It is, of course, to be hoped that the board will have a continuing interest in the department, but it need not enter directly into the administration. Reference to the relationship of hospital trustees and the department is made in Chapter 14, "People and Problems." The architect also has done his part and need not continue except to fulfill his contract by assuring that everything he recommended is working properly.

In the author's opinion, responsibility for the day-to-day operation of the department is better assumed by an individual than by a group. For this reason a director of the emergency department is recommended. He must be a doctor, and it is to be preferred that he participate in the actual care of patients. He must, however, have some place to turn for support and advice, and some responsible group must make sure he is directing. The author's experience with job descriptions and intricate tables of organization has led him to believe that they have some, but limited, value. Some people take them too seriously and as a result either use them to overstep reason or, just as bad, as a refuge from failure to carry responsibility. Someone has aptly stated, "We must have standards from which to deviate." The same may be said about job descriptions and tables of organization. Whatever the decision is with regard to responsibility and channels of authority, there should be a doctor of medicine at the head of an emergency department. He should have conferred on him, by either the hospital or the medical staff bylaws, the authority to make and enforce decisions when prompt action is called for. His authority should not be diluted by a maze of solid or broken lines in a table of organization, indicating that he cannot issue orders to certain personnel in the department. He should be captain of the ship.

Considering the amount of work done there, the exposure of the department to public scrutiny and criticism, and the necessity for constant cooperation with and by major clinical departments of the hospital, the head of the department has the same right to serve on the executive committee of the medical staff as has any other department chief. He should be a party to decisions that affect the functioning of his department. This, however, does not obviate the necessity for an emergency department committee with membership as suggested above.

SIZE OF THE COMMITTEE

It is a mistake to have too large a committee. It has been the author's observation that entirely too many large com-

mittees are appointed around hospitals. This puts too great
a burden on some members of the medical staff. In one hospital where he was well acquainted with the medical staff
organization he noted that one member was serving on nine
committees, several were serving on seven or eight, and quite
a number on six. In a large staff, talent is not so scarce as to
justify this. A committee of three to five people who have
sufficient interest to study and work on problems is far more
effective than one of eight to twelve, with some members
giving no thought to the problems between committee meetings. The M.D. director of the department should serve on
the committee as should one but no more than two other
doctors. One nurse is enough, and she should probably represent a higher position than the chief nurse of the emergency
department. The latter may be invited to any meetings where
her functions and responsibilities are to be discussed. Administration should be represented, for recommendations of this
committee often involve administrative decisions. This is
enough. The inviting of noncommittee members to meet with
the committee when their skills or knowledge are required is
a good pattern to follow, but there is no value in naming a
person to a committee just so a certain group will be represented.

An important fact, yet one often forgotten by some doctors,
is that no portion of the whole hospital program is exclusively
medical. Wise is the hospital administrator who refrains from
taking stands or expressing opinions in matters purely medical,
but few purely medical activities go on around a hospital that
are not dependent on administrative support. This goes beyond
matters of money, although this is one area where doctors may
need understanding and sympathetic restraint. Many hospital
administrators have a fairly good knowledge of the law as it
applies to hospital practice. They almost always have an appreciation of public relations, and they do or should have an
idea of how the governing board is likely to view changes in
policy. Here again is an area where some doctors find it difficult
to understand their relationships to hospitals. What they do
in the treatment of their own private patients is for them to

decide as long as it is not in conflict with good medical practice and the bylaws the medical staff has adopted. When matters of overall hospital policy are concerned, however, they must bow to the decisions of the governing board as interpreted to them by administration. The law has stated and, more and more, is restating that the governing board is responsible for what goes on in the hospital.

This matter of the position of administration and medical staff has a very direct bearing on the directorship of the emergency department. If the department is staffed by hospital-salaried doctors including the director, the administration has a major responsibility in the selection of and in the supervision of the director. If these doctors are all in private practice on a fee-for-service basis, the administrator has less responsibility and authority over them. The director may have his duties and responsibilities so defined as to partly stem from hospital administration and partly from the medical staff. This dual position has hazards that must be recognized before it is entered into. The author feels strongly that the professional activities of the doctors practicing in the emergency department should be subject to the same type of control exercised by the medical staff elsewhere in the hospital. This is the only way that the quality of work there can be kept at a high level. However, if these doctors are in private practice and subject to the rules and regulations of the medical staff, they have an equal right to full representation on the executive committee of the medical staff. Medical staffs, where the executive committee is made up of staff officers and department chiefs, are downgrading the importance of emergency department practice if they do not give the emergency department director equal status with other chiefs or chairmen. The problems are too acute to be handled through third-party reports. The director should have direct access to the executive committee so that he may explain his problems and proposed solutions.

The administration of an emergency department carries with it community responsibility. Demographic studies of the community are important to any phase of health-care planning. Any agency or group participating in such planning is shortsighted if it does not take into consideration the composition and shifting of the population in a nation that is evolving as rapidly as is the United States. However, certain fundamentals, so evident as to need no defense, must be recognized and must remain as bases from which to work. One of these is that whether the population is static or has a rapid turnover, accidents and other emergencies do not change as far as they require medical and surgical management. They call for planning that will provide prompt, high-grade diagnosis and treatment. The desire of a shifting population to have centers to which it can repair for all types of medical attention should in no way be allowed to alter the plans for this prompt, high-grade emergency care. Unfortunately, some planners have been influenced by pressure from this shifting population, and emergency care has suffered from their shortsightedness. Under the guise of facing reality, they have actually retreated from it. It is the responsibility of these planners to provide other facilities for these people who depend on the hospital rather than on physicians for total medical care. Means to this end are discussed in Chapter 21, "Emergency Department vs Outpatient Department."

Since the patient who comes to the hospital emergency department receives services from two sources—the physician and the hospital, the responsibilities of the two must be considered separately. The physician has the responsibility, when he accepts the patient, to provide medical or surgical care on a level with standard accepted practice. The law no longer limits this to a level of practice customary in the community. Physicians are constantly reminded of this as they see or hear about their colleagues becoming involved in litigation. They protect their interests by insurance against malpractice, although it is well known that careful examination, accurate diagnosis, good treatment, and full and honest records are the best protection against such action.

The service provided by the hospital is the responsibility of the governing board and the administrator is its agent. For that reason, he has the responsibility to provide a high standard of service. This involves equipment, supplies, and personnel.

With this responsibility should go administrative authority, and in certain areas this may overlap the authority of the doctors. For instance, insofar as the hospital is liable to litigation, the administrator has the right to insist on practices that will not jeopardize the hospital. One of these is the matter of records. It is the doctor's responsibility to write the record or to have it written for his approval and signature. Since in the course of his examination and treatment he is using hospital facilities and personnel, the hospital (the administrator) has the right to insist that he record accurately what was done. Hospital administrators have no hesitancy in demanding complete records on inpatients. It is just as imperative that they demand the same standards on outpatients. This includes completeness and promptness. The latter is sometimes more necessary here than in the wards or in the operating room. These treatments are one-shot affairs, and the recording cannot be left to a more convenient day. Of course, it is to be hoped that the medical records department and the medical records committee will so carry their responsibilities that no administrative urging will be required.

So we see that an unwritten table of organization and an acceptable chain of command are essential to the production of standard or superior emergency department patient care. The governing board is responsible for this quality. It depends on the administrator to represent it and carry out its wishes. The medical staff and the nursing service must provide the actual care. The on-the-spot supervision, as well as some of the actual care, will be the responsibility of the director, who will have full authority. He, however, must have the support and, where needed, the guidance of a multidisciplined committee capable of understanding all the problems of the department. Estimates of the quality of the service must be provided through periodic reviews, involving both doctors and nurses. Reference to such self-examination by those working in an emergency department in a New Jersey hospital will be found in Chapter 19, "Evaluation." The director of surgery in that hospital told the author that in their first review, which followed a survey by a team of surgeons from other hospitals, they brought to light what they classified as several avoidable fatalities. The death audit program,[2] which is enjoying wide acceptance in hospital practice, is easily adapted to emergency department practice.

Since the physical facilities of no department of a hospital remain in optimum working condition, it is the responsibility of administration to delegate periodic maintenance. In Chapter 5, mention is made of frequent (daily) testing of such items as the defibrillator. This is an administrative responsibility but carried out by those actively using the equipment. Reports on such tests should be included in the reports of the director to the executive committee of the medical staff. Where the hoped-for *esprit de corps* exists in the department, everyone will strive for excellence, and the authority provided to get these things done will seldom need to be in evidence. This *esprit de corps* is quite likely to stem from the top and is the result of under-standing cooperation coupled with well-executed authority. A young assistant hospital administrator stated that the head of the university department where he got his degree once asked the class what was the most important thing for a hospital administrator to strive for. None of the answers satisfied him. The answer he wanted was "survival." This story was told at a luncheon honoring an administrator who had just completed a quarter century of service in one hospital. He still held the respect and admiration of nearly everyone with whom he worked, even though on many occasions he had differed with them. I could not help but compare this record with that of another administrator who was removed by a lethargic govern-ing board, but only after the doctors said they could take no more.

REFERENCES

1. Hawley, P.R.: Personal communication.
2. Snedecor, S.T.: Could your emergency department save seriously in-jured patients? *Bull Am Coll Surgeons,* 52:275–277, 1967.

Chapter 9

COOPERATION WITH OTHER DEPARTMENTS

Although we have stated that the emergency facility deserves departmental status (if it is properly planned and operated), it must be borne in mind that this department cannot function without close cooperation with certain other hospital departments. It is quite evident that the medical staff, the nursing service, and administration are all part of the makeup of the emergency department. However, it is dependent on certain services from the department of laboratories and the department of radiology and cannot function without them. Indeed, assistance from these departments, particularly x-ray, is needed daily. The incidence of fractures among patients appearing at the emergency department makes the x-ray department indispensable.

The department of anesthesia also renders essential support in many emergency departments.

LABORATORY

In the largest hospitals, where the emergency department is comprehensive and has a large, full-time, around-the-clock staff, there may be a clinical laboratory physically within the department. If so, this will function entirely as a support of the emergency department, but even then it will probably be staffed by and controlled by the laboratory department of the hospital. Emergency cases during their stay in the emergency department seldom require intricate laboratory determinations or for that matter, many laboratory determinations. However, such things as hematocrits, hemoglobin determinations, blood counts, certain urinalyses, and other tests are frequently necessary. A working arrangement must be made with the department of laboratories to supply these services as needed. The arrangement must provide prompt laboratory service. This can result in differences of opinion to the point of friction, but it need not. Well-function-

159

ing laboratories are used to emergency requests from elsewhere in the hospital and will respond to such requests from the emergency department provided the groundwork has been laid.

Having a small laboratory where hemoglobins and urinalyses and other simple tests can be done by a nurse in charge or by the doctor will relieve the regular laboratory personnel from unnecessary night calls. On the other hand, certain cases will call for hematocrit determinations, and often these will need to be repeated from time to time. When they are needed, they are needed promptly. Quick blood-sugar determinations are needed in suspected cases of diabetic coma or insulin shock. There are other situations where the treatment of the patient cannot be decided upon until reports are available from the laboratory. Severely injured patients in shock will frequently require blood transfusion while in the emergency department. This will, of course, require typing, and it is much safer to have this done by laboratory technicians who are doing it constantly, than it is for a nurse or a doctor to do it occasionally. Blood-gas studies and other more sophisticated tests may sometimes be indicated, particularly in shock patients.

Unless the laboratory technicians are actually on duty at night or at other off-hours, those responsible for patients in the emergency department should intelligently plan the laboratory work as needed and order it promptly so that, if necessary, several tests may be done at the same time. Nothing is more provoking to a laboratory technician who has already done a long day's work and who must necessarily be up early the next morning than to have an emergency department doctor vacillate about what he needs until the technician is about to go back to bed, and then decide that he had better have other tests which could just as well have been ordered an hour before. These are all matters of consideration for the rights and comforts of others and, of course, should be expected in all interdepartmental relations throughout the hospital.

X-RAY

A properly motivated x-ray department will recognize true emergencies and will give them a higher priority than their routine work. Granted that it is disturbing to have to take x-rays of a fractured femur just at the time when it was planned to begin a gastrointestinal series, there is no question that the femur should come first. On the other hand, if a physician sends in a patient who he thought yesterday had a sprained ankle but to-day thinks may have a fractured fibula, there is no reason why a G.I. series should be held up until the ankle is x-rayed. Here again, it is a matter of putting first things first and recognizing true emergencies. The time to reduce a fracture which has oc-curred within the last hour or two is right now. The x-ray diag-nosis should be made available as rapidly as possible.

It is necessary here to warn against unfairness to x-ray tech-nicians at night and during off-hours. It would be difficult to justify getting an x-ray technician out of bed to take x-rays at midnight on an extremity that was injured 24 to 48 hours ago. The optimum time for reduction, if needed, has now passed. If information regarding the types of injuries to patients coming to the hospital is available ahead of time, it is frequently possible to summon the x-ray technician and have him or her waiting when the patient arrives. When ambulance service is well co-ordinated with the hospital, frequently the reports sent in either by telephone or two-way radio will alert the emergency depart-ment staff to fractures so that the x-ray department may be notified. Again the emergency department staff should plan to order all of the x-rays needed as promptly as possible so that the technicians may proceed to take the films and not wait for a while and have to take others. Where there are fractures requir-ing reduction, conscientious x-ray personnel will gladly wait until after the reduction is accomplished to take postreduction films. On the other hand, where there are fractures with no displace-ment whatsoever, but still requiring a cast, there is no necessity for requiring a technician to remain for a half-hour to an hour while the cast is applied, in order to take a postcast film that will show nothing not visible on the original. This is not to say that follow-up films should not be taken, but there is no necessity for taking them in the middle of the night when this causes further loss of sleep by the x-ray department personnel.

Most physicians capable of caring for fractures will be able to read their own x-rays, and it is seldom necessary to call the radiologist during the night. However, if there are problems of difficulty in reading films and where the accurate x-ray diagnosis will influence emergency treatment, there should be no hesitancy in asking the radiologist to come to the hospital and render his opinion. After all, he is a physician, and this aspect of the patient's care is his responsibility.

There should be a standing rule that no one in the x-ray department may remove a splint without authorization from the treating physician.

DEPARTMENT OF ANESTHESIA

The problem of general anesthesia is a major one. As Shortliffe[1] observes, "There is no such thing as a minor general anesthetic." We must go further. There is no such thing as minor surgery under a general anesthetic. The elements that make surgery major or minor are the elements of danger—danger to life or danger of disability. The anesthesia and the operation should be considered together in estimating the risk and, of course, the patient's condition must be included. Many emergency department patients requiring general anesthesia for surgery are not as good surgical risks as those prepared for scheduled elective operations.

The decision about general anesthesia and surgery requiring it in the emergency department must follow a frank answer to the question, "Will our equipment, our personnel, and our attitude provide as safe treatment as if it were done in the regular operating room?" If the answer is positive, then the decision is one to be based on convenience.

The safety of the patient who receives a general anesthetic in the emergency department is the dual responsibility of the emergency department and the department of anesthesia. The acceptance of this responsibility is essential to good patient care. It must never be forgotten, however, that in the final analysis, the responsibility for the patient's treatment (and this includes all phases) and the patient's safety lies with the primary treating physician.

OTHER DEPARTMENTS

Certain associations with other departments are necessary, but these are, for the most part, not as intimate as those with the laboratory, x-ray, and anesthesia departments. There may be times when the dietary department may be asked to provide nourishment for patients being detained overnight or for some hours in one of the holding beds, or there may be times when the emergency department staff, working long hours, may need food. There should be no difficulty in working out a plan of smooth cooperation.

One authority has suggested that the intensive care unit of the hospital should be constructed near the emergency department. This would be a splendid arrangement if thought were being given only to emergency department patients, but it would probably not meet with the approval of administration, surgical staff, or various others concerned with the care of acutely ill patients. Whereas an intensive care unit could function as an extension of the emergency department, the average intensive care unit is more likely to be fed from the operating rooms and by direct admission than from the emergency department, and consequently it is better located near surgery and, as it frequently is, near or in conjunction with the recovery room. Not only will the surgeons and the anesthesiologists want to have it close at hand where they can see patients but so will the internists for their acutely ill patients. In the very small hospital where there is not sufficient personnel and equipment to keep a well-organized emergency department, recovery room, and intensive care unit functioning separately, it may be advantageous to have these all close together. In one 60-bed hospital where the author visited the emergency department as a member of a survey team, he found it right next door to the recovery room, and as this hospital did not have an intensive care unit, it could have been considered that the functions of the intensive care unit were covered by the combined emergency and recovery rooms. This was a satisfactory arrangement in this institution of limited personnel and equipment, but under ordinary circumstances, the intensive care unit should be located where it will best serve the entire hospital rather than where it will bolster up the service of the emergency department. As a matter of fact, a properly staffed emergency department, which includes in its facilities some observation beds, is in truth an intensive care unit.

It scarcely seems necessary to add that the emergency department should have a good working arrangement with central supply. Unless the department is large enough to justify its own supply room complete with sterilizing equipment, such as seen at the Radcliffe Infirmary, Oxford, England, the Birmingham Accident Hospital, and many of our larger institutions, it will be dependent on central supply daily. The placing of responsibility and authority should be such that at no time will the emergency department be handicapped by a shortage of supplies, including sterile items.

There is no better way to judge the professional atmosphere of a hospital than to observe the cooperation between departments discussed here. Where the cooperation is friendly and smooth, patients are most likely to receive superior care.

REFERENCE

1. Shortliffe, E.C.: Emergency department. Some considerations on physical facilities. *Hospitals,* 36:48–125 *passim,* 1962.

Chapter 10

MEDICAL RECORDS

The author was invited to address the American Association of Medical Record Librarians when it met in Chicago in 1963. Following my talk, I moderated a discussion period. I have seldom had the privilege of talking with a group of people in the health field with so much interest in and knowledge of its specialty. My formal remarks,* with slight modifications, follow.

The finest dietary department, the cleanest laundry, the most fireproof building, and modern operating rooms do not guarantee good patient care, but in the medical records it is pretty difficult to consistently cover up bad care. When the medical staff is doing a good job in diagnosis and treatment, the records show it. If it isn't, the records will tell the story.

If I were asked to evaluate a hospital and then told that I could visit only one department in making this evaluation, I would unhesitatingly choose the record room. Only in the record room could I attempt to judge patient care, and patient care is the purpose of the hospital.

In the days before the American College of Surgeons turned over the survey and approval of hospitals to the Joint Commission on Accreditation of Hospitals, the point system was used in rating a hospital. A completely satisfactory report on every phase of hospital organization and operation netted the hospital 1000 points. The highest number of points was allotted to medical staff organization and medical records.

I would never suggest that any doctor, nurse, aid, or orderly neglect for a moment the actual care of a patient in order to keep a good record, but pre-emergency planning can usually

* These remarks were reprinted and circulated to administrators of Ontario hospitals by the Ontario Hospital Association.

result in the combined achievement of good care and an accurate record.

It is in this pre-emergency planning that the medical record librarian can be of inestimable value. She knows, better than anyone else, the embarrassments that may arise from inadequate emergency department records. No emergency department committee should be named without including a representative from the medical records department or, at least, without providing for consultation with that department.

The physician thinks he knows what he wants in the record for future reference in follow-up care, and the nurse thinks she knows what she wants—to be able to report just what she observed and what she did—but it is the medical record librarian who really knows what information doctors, nurses, administrators, lawyers, and insurance representatives look for when they consult these records a week or a year later.

The reasons for accurate and complete medical records in general all apply to emergency department records, but some reasons need more emphasis in this phase of hospital activity. They may be grouped under litigation, aid in patient care, and review or evaluation of care given in the emergency department.

IN LITIGATION, RECORDS PROTECT ALL

Since emergency situations often involve legal responsibility, almost anyone who takes part in the production of the situation or in handling it may become involved in litigation when it ensues.

This fact provides the first sound argument for good records. This argument has three facets: protection of the physician and the hospital, of the patient, and of the individual alleged to be responsible for the emergency.

If the emergency situation involves an injury, as it often does, the injured person usually feels that someone is to blame for this. When the subjects of expense, loss of time, and temporary or permanent disability come up, he feels that someone else should pay. If he doesn't arrive at this conclusion by his own mental processes, he may be aided in his thinking by disinterested or, more likely, interested parties.

First he blames and possibly sues the party responsible for the accident. Then if things aren't going well, he may decide that the doctor or the hospital has not given him proper treatment and is to some degree responsible for his incomplete recovery. Again, he may have aid in arriving at this conclusion. He sues.

In my years of practice I always tried to keep good medical records and, at times, made myself unpopular by insisting that others do the same. My motivation, however, was not fear of suit. I always had the feeling that if a physician kept informed of modern trends in treatment and used these with discretion, he was in little danger from malpractice suits. I felt the same way about hospitals. That some of the new weapons in the armamentarium of the physician and surgeon have increased his exposure to legal risks cannot be doubted. The use of some of these weapons involves a calculated risk, and when he takes that risk he is well advised to record accurately why he is doing it and how. This record may save him embarrassment, not to mention his livelihood.

Good records in the emergency department are also needed for the protection of the patient. When someone else is responsible for his misfortune and he seeks redress, he may be well within his rights. An accurate and complete record of his injuries and his general condition when he arrived at the emergency department of the hospital is basic to his case. His response to treatment at the time and as the situation progresses, as well as a fair estimate of the ultimate result, is equally important. A comparison of his physical state and his abilities before and after his misfortune may be aided by a few intelligently recorded notes on his record.

INCLUDING DEFENDANT

The third facet of the litigation argument for good emergency department records is the protection of the defendant or, if he is insured, his insurance carrier. This feature might fairly be called the protection of the public, for directly or indirectly the public will sooner or later pay the award. I regret having to make this statement, and I would not have made it in my early years of practice, but I am convinced that because of today's mores, the defendant and his insurance carrier need help to a greater degree than does the plaintiff. This conclusion, for which I take full responsibility, is based on several observations.

Over the years and in increasing numbers of cases, I have seen the seriousness and importance of injuries magnified beyond all reason when litigation has become a factor. I will not point the finger of accusation directly at anyone, but I must add that I don't believe this situation usually stems from greed or dishonesty on the part of the injured person. Sometimes it does but more often not. Third parties play a part, and they aren't always lawyers.

One of the most blatant of these situations arose in my own family. One of my brothers, his wife, and daughter were involved in an automobile accident in Massachusetts. The injuries were not great, but the wife and daughter were in the hospital two or three days. I went to see them and assured myself that recovery would be prompt and complete.

The other driver's insurance company offered my brother $2000 and complete repair of his car. Being a college professor, this was more money than he had ever seen. He asked my advice and said a nurse had told him to demand $5000 and get a lawyer. I told him to forget the lawyer and take the $2000 before the man changed his mind. I think they painted their house, bought some household appliances, and put a nice amount in the bank—from the insurance check.

I have seen injured patients retarded in their recovery, or at least in evidence of recovery, while they waited their turn in the court room where their unreasonable demands would be settled. I have seen them recover rapidly after what has been aptly called the application of the "green poultice."

I have also seen them come out of the small end of the horn, by failing to get their demands and by incurring legal expenses which resulted in much less in pocket than would a just settlement offered by a reputable insurance company. They have been victimized by their own greed and stupidity.

If we are interested in reason and justice, complete, accurate, and honest emergency room records may aid in getting it. This is particularly true where impartial medical testimony is practiced.

RECORDS AID IN PATIENT CARE

The record of examination, diagnosis, and treatment in the emergency department is of great value to the treating physician in the following hours and days if he continues to be responsible for the care of the patient, either after admission to the hospital or in his office. This record is of even greater value to another physician who did not see the patient in the emergency department, if said patient is to continue under his care, either as an inpatient or an outpatient.

If the injury was a laceration of the scalp and the patient was admitted after treatment, it isn't enough for the physician to whom the patient is referred to be told, "Oh, Joe, I admitted a guy last night after I sewed up his scalp." The second physician should know how long and how deep the laceration was and if the wound was dirty. He should know if the wound was debrided and irrigated before suture. He should know if cranial or intracranial damage is suspected and if x-rays were taken and what they showed. He should know if tetanus immunization was started. He should have all available information to make the care he gives the patient rational and effective.

AND IN EVALUATION OF EMERGENCY DEPARTMENT

The third supporting reason for maintaining good records in the emergency department is their use in evaluating the department itself. Several agencies or groups are interested in such evaluation. These include the American College of Surgeons, the Joint Commission on Accreditation of Hospitals, the medical staff, the nursing administration, and the hospital administration.

Mention has been made in the chapter on evaluation of

emergency departments of the interest the American College of Surgeons has taken in this. The studies could not have been made without at least fairly good records. This is particularly true in the study reported by Skudder,[1] "An Experiment in Evaluating the Management of Trauma." In this report, Skudder points out some of the deficiencies in emergency department records.

The Joint Commission on Accreditation of Hospitals includes the emergency department in its hospital survey program. As the overall theme of the accreditation program is better and safer patient care, the Commission concerns itself with activities here and depends among other things on the emergency department records to substantiate the quality of care given.

PUT IN SUMMARIES AS WELL AS CASES

No medical staff really desiring to provide the best possible care for the hospital patient will fail to voluntarily review its failures and successes. These failures and successes are not limited to the care of the individual patient but involve the functioning of departments and programs. Evaluation of the type and quality of work done in the emergency department must of necessity be based on records kept. These include not only the individual case records but also periodic summaries of them. Weekly or monthly reports prepared by an emergency department nurse or some other responsible person should include such data as the following: number of visits; classification as to true emergencies; breakdown into medical, surgical, obstetrical, and other classifications; number of fractures treated and whether they were open or closed; number of anesthesias given; number of poison cases, when the department functions as a "poison center"; and other statistical data which may be requested by the administrator, chief nurse, or medical staff.

Such a report from the emergency department should stimulate staff members to evaluate the quality as well as the quantity of the work accomplished there. This report should not be used merely to satisfy some requirement.

It might suggest the need for trauma or fracture conferences where staff members could improve their knowledge and techniques and thus upgrade the quality of patient care. A little imagination on the part of the person who prepares the report would make it not only valuable but stimulating.

A staff member wanting to make a study of his or the department's results in the care of certain types of cases, particularly in the field of trauma, would find good emergency department records a fertile source of information.

The nursing administration would find such records invaluable in planning nursing service for the department and equipping it with supplies.

Finally, the administrator, seeking to be sure that the emergency department is fulfilling to the best of its ability its obligation to the community, would want to know the amount of and type of patient care provided there. Requests to him for added or altered facilities should be supported by records proving the need. Seen from any angle, an emergency department is no better than its records.

WHO IS RESPONSIBLE FOR RECORDS?

Assuming that the need for adequate emergency room records has been established, who is responsible for them? Responsibility of this kind cannot be placed on certain people: it belongs to a certain person. That person is the doctor who examines and treats the patient.

The patient may not be clear in his mind as to what he is seeking when he comes to the emergency room. Many come to the hospital because they think the hospital will treat them. It won't. The doctor will. While the hospital helps him by means of nursing and laboratory service and equipment, only he is going to make the diagnosis, plan the treatment, and apply it, or at least supervise it. Briefly, the doctor calls the shots. For that reason, the record is his responsibility. He may not actually write everything that goes on the chart. He may dictate it or allow someone else to fill it in, but he is responsible for it and should approve and sign it.

He may delegate, but he may not abdicate.

Now let us consider the form for such a record. Let us consider this against the background of the mournful wail about records in general. Everyone has heard these wails. My voice has joined the lament, and yet I have argued for good medical records and have tried to keep them.

Have you ever seen a physician on the witness stand sweating under pressure because the medical record in his hand is incomplete? I have.

Have you ever seen a doctor presenting a case report at a staff meeting become embarrassed because he couldn't find some essential detail in his record? I have.

These things can be obviated by good record forms—if the doctors will use them.

FORM MUST BE A GUIDE

It has been said that the best medical record form is a blank sheet of 8½″ x 11″ paper. This is not true. A rare physician might, in most cases, record on such a sheet all the essential data to identify his patient, describe his medical history, indicate his physical condition, substantiate his diagnosis, defend his therapeutic regimen, and verify the end result, but he wouldn't always do it. To gather together a group of such physicians to staff a hospital would be impossible. No, we need forms. They must be guides that will assure complete and standardized data.

Opinions will differ as to what constitutes essential data on emergency department forms, but certain principles should be universally accepted.

These forms should be
  1. Complete.
  2. Concise, yet with essential details.
  3. Easy to read.
  4. Easy to fill out.

They should contain
  Essential details—administrative.

1. Identification.
2. Parent or other sponsor (if a minor).
3. Employer (if responsible).
4. Witnesses (to accident).
5. Brought by.
6. Financial responsibility.

Essential details—clinical.

1. History—short but accurate (blank space or lined).
2. Physical examination—brief but informative.
3. Diagnosis—detailed.
   a. Lacerations—location and length.
   b. Abrasions or contusions—location.
   c. Burns—location, size, degree.
   d. Fractures or dislocations (use accepted terminology).
4. Treatment—brief.
   a. Fractures—x-ray, reduction, cast.
   b. Sutures—number.
   c. Medication.
   d. Anesthesia.

They should establish

Financial responsibility.

1. Personal—always.
2. Insurance—if covered.

   a. Blue Cross.
      (1) Name of plan.
      (2) Policy number.
   b. Blue Shield.
      (1) Name of plan.
      (2) Policy number.
   c. Other carriers.
      (1) Name and address.
      (2) Policy number.

Insurance forms should be available.

They should be

Color-coded (at least three copies) for

1. Emergency department file.

2. Patient's chart (if admitted).
3. Treating physician.

Finally, they should
  Encourage.
    1. Completeness.
    2. Legibility.
    3. Promptness.
  Discourage.
    1. Abbreviations.
    2. Colloquialisms.
    3. Carelessness.

AFTER EMERGENCY DEPARTMENT, WHERE TO?

Disposition of the patient when he leaves the emergency department should be a part of the record. It should indicate whether he is

1. Admitted to the hospital.
2. Referred to his private physician.
3. Followed up for further care by treating physician.
4. Referred to the outpatient department.
5. Subject to other disposition.

Disposition, it should be observed here, should not only be on the record, but should be made clear to the patient or his family. Any follow-up instructions regarding care at home should be made clear. To avoid misunderstanding, instructions may best be put in writing. Some hospitals request the patient to sign a statement that he has been so instructed, and forms for this should be available.

Of course, forms for written permission to give an anesthetic or carry out any but the simplest surgical procedure should be available. Forms for release from responsibility to be signed when patients refuse treatment will protect both hospital and doctor. This is discussed in the chapter on people and problems.

USE A LITTLE TIME TO SAVE A LOT OF TIME

It is advisable to keep in the emergency departments the standard report forms for the Blue Cross and Blue Shield Plans that cover patients in the community. Forms from commercial insurance companies which insure sizable numbers of people in the community are also useful. A little time spent completing these forms may save a lot of time later. This can be done in a manner that will not appear mercenary. In fact, many patients appreciate it.

Instructions regarding the completion of the emergency department forms should be posted in the department. To avoid any misunderstanding, these should be agreed to by the staff so that a nurse who has to urge a doctor to complete the form will be backed by staff authority.

Attention to details is a prerequisite to good medical care and accurate forms stress this. Good medical records are inseparable from good medical care. They are part of it.

REFERENCE

1. Skudder, P.A.: An experiment in evaluating the management of trauma. *Bull Am Coll Surgeons*, 46:42–43, 65–67, 1961.

Chapter 11

HOSPITAL DISASTER PLANS

Whether the emergency department will be the nerve center of the hospital disaster plan will depend largly on its physical arrangement. If Amspacher[1] is right, it cannot be. He stated, "A hospital has an emergency room of some type. It will usually be a cut-up affair which will need to be abandoned immediately and some of the best parts of the hospital will need to be taken over as an admitting ward." Architects' plans for emergency departments, sometimes seen, immediately rule out such departments as the initial area to which mass casualties may be admitted. If it is true that an open treatment area is more practical for the treating of a half-dozen injured people than is a row of six small rooms, then this is even more important when many more injured are admitted. A large treatment area coupled with a sizeable waiting room from which the furniture may be quickly removed might make the emergency department the best sorting or triage area in the hospital. It has the advantage, of course, of being well equipped and stocked with supplies. If the structure of the department is such as to disqualify it for consideration as a sorting area, other space must be so designated in the disaster plan. This may be a large ground floor dining room or other space where multiple stretchers may be placed.

The author discussed the subject of disaster plans in an address delivered at the Woman's Medical College, Philadelphia, during a symposium on civil defense. This was sponsored by the MEND program. The address is reproduced here with minor alterations.[2]

MASS CASUALTIES IN THE CIVILIAN HOSPITAL

The care of mass casualties involves a professional philosophy distinct from that followed in the private practice of medicine. It may be summarized as pointing toward the greatest good for the greatest number. Whether the cause of the casualties is enemy action or other disaster, the plan for their care requires predisaster thinking, if confusion and chaos are to be avoided.

The motto of the Medical Department of the United States Army is "to conserve fighting strength," the implication of course being that the primary mission is not to make sick and wounded soldiers well so they can return home, but so they can fight again. It was my observation during a tour of active duty in World War II that medical officers who were able to rationalize and embrace that approach to military medicine were much happier and more effective than those motivated only by the humanitarian approach. This did not mean that they had to be callous or unsympathetic, but it did mean that they had to put the interest of the greatest number foremost. At times they had to abandon critically injured men who had little chance of survival in order to care for others who might survive as the results of their efforts.

Plan Is Preventive Medicine

It would be foolhardy for me to try to predict how any of us would react, if we were able to react, to an all-out thermonuclear attack. However, it is not foolhardy for us to plan what we would do if a tornado rips through our area leaving desolation in its wake, or if a factory containing explosives blows up, or two passenger trains collide at high speed, or even if we find ourselves in the fringes of an enemy attack and still alive and able to use our training among the survivors. Predisaster planning is simply a phase of preventive medicine, and the physician or hospital administrator who turns up his nose at it puts himself in the same category as the parent who refuses immunization for his child because he "doesn't believe in shots."

With this appeal to you to see this problem in the light of the ever present thought that "it might happen to us," let me go on to a working definition of mass casualties. To me this term means a sudden concentration of casualties that overwhelms the existing medical facilities. This may be a group of victims from a two-car crash, with one driver having a crushed chest with pneumothorax and a fractured femur, a passenger with a fractured pelvis and a ruptured bladder, two with head injuries producing coma, and three others suffering from multiple fractures and profound shock. Such a catastrophe in a rural area with only one physician, however capable, constitutes mass casualties.

On the other hand, the term would apply to the victims of an explosion in a plant manufacturing a highly inflammable product which suddenly presents a swarm of severely burned and otherwise critically injured people at the emergency entrance of a well-organized and staffed metropolitan hospital. The rural physician might, by superhuman effort and in a minimum of time, introduce a catheter into the chest of the driver victim and institute underwater seal drainage, direct that a Thomas splint with moderate traction be put on the femur, get a catheter into the ruptured bladder, do a tracheostomy on one of the head victims showing respiratory distress, direct infusion of dextran for the three shock victims as well as the application of splints to reduce further shock, provided the physician had in his little hospital one or two good orderlies and some nurses who knew how to take and *record* blood pressures and insert intravenous needles. If he did all these things well enough and soon enough, he might then have seven living patients showing enough improvement to justify more deliberate evaluation, and he could then plan his priorities for definitive treatment and summon whatever professional assistance he might need. I can assure you, however, that unless he had pictured himself in such a situation before and made some plan of attack, he wouldn't get all these things done well enough and soon enough, and he wouldn't have seven live patients.

Disaster Plan Necessary

I can also assure you that the metropolitan hospital with the mass admission of explosion victims is going to experience a fairly high mortality if thought has not been given to more than adequate dressings, plasma volume expanders, and other supplies, and a workable and rehearsed plan of getting its medical staff out of its offices or off the golf courses and off-duty nurses back on duty. The plan must provide for the sudden conversion of a smoothly working general hospital into a cross between a collecting station and an evacuation hospital. I well remember seeing 525 men from a troopship torpedoed in the English Channel admitted to a military hospital in Cherbourg on Christmas Eve in 1944. Seeing extra cots taken out of storage and set up in predetermined areas as if this were an everyday practice astounded the commanding general of Normandy Base Section. Being a line officer, he did not expect such precision from the medical department. He spoke to me about this, but I didn't tell him that sometime previously, all available space in that hospital had been measured and a pattern plotted for the extra cots. We hadn't expected a sudden influx of patients from the Channel, but we had been told that we might without much warning get large numbers of casualties from the opposite direction.

Quality of Care Dependent on Planning and Discipline

The quality of care of large numbers of injured patients in any hospital will depend to a great extent on predisaster planning and on the degree of cooperation shown by all echelons of hospital personnel. A plan that will not break down under pressure presupposes authority and discipline. Many human beings find it easy to submit to these, but some do not. Probably a higher percentage of this latter class may be found among physicians than among other groups of hospital workers. These individuals must be dealt with carefully in order that their talents may be used to the fullest, but there must be a limit to how much they are coddled.

When a hospital disaster-plan committee sits down to assign duties to medical staff members, there is more to consider than medical skills. Personalities and past behavior may well be considered. The job to which a physician is assigned may strike him as beneath his dignity. If so, make a change, but this time make the assignment stick. Keep in mind that calm judgment is as important as technical skill when the pressure is on. Let the prima donnas work in the operating room, if they are capable, but don't forget to hold out one or more experienced surgeons for the sorting department. It is here that the big decisions are made and the priorities established.

The Disaster Plan

Space for the reception of new patients in large numbers is a problem that must be solved and may well be the first item on the agenda of the disaster plan committee. Just as military hospitals along the line extending from the battle area to the rear must have a plan of evacuation to clear space for new casualties, so the civilian hospital should incorporate the same feature in its mass casualty plan. When the situation requires the admission of numbers of patients far beyond the usual capacity of the hospital, some of the existing patients must be discharged immediately. The responsibility for this should be assigned to a member or members of the medical staff with sufficient aid from the nursing staff. This is no time to keep in the hospital ambulatory medical cases, partially convalesced ambulatory surgical cases, and certainly not patients in for so-called "clinical study." Decisions on these discharges must be intelligent but prompt. A mild air of martial law must prevail. Most patients will be cooperative. Those who are not must be dealt with kindly but firmly. This is no time to think about possible lawsuits. No court of law that deserves any respect would recognize such claims in the face of a pressing disaster.

Space must be prepared for the care of incoming patients so that clogging of the stream of traffic does not occur. If time permits, these evacuated patients should be given discharge instructions, particularly with regard to getting in contact with their private physicians or the hospital clinic when the emergency is over. Such instructions may be given on prepared forms.

Liaison with local civil defense authorities will strengthen a hospital disaster plan, as the transportation of injured people to the hospital may well be under the direction of such authorities. The hospital itself has a responsibility outside the building, however, as the approach to the hospital emergency entrance is of primary importance. I can think of two large city hospitals, one of them connected with a leading medical school, where I hope no large convoy of ambulances or other vehicles has to unload in a hurry, unless their approaches are modified. Both have a bottleneck entrance to the emergency department which would require the most expert traffic control to prevent a serious traffic snarl. Situations of this kind indicate a blind spot in the thinking of the architects or administrators of these hospitals.

In the type of world in which we live today, no hospital is completely fulfilling its obligation to the community if it is not able to receive large numbers of patients at one time with a minimum of confusion. This requires easy entrance to and exit from the unloading area.

Many hospitals, without prohibitive expenditures, would be unable to provide space under their roofs for the prompt reception of overwhelming numbers of patients, but plans should be made for a sorting area under canvas, in a garage or laundry, or in some other way that ingenuity might prescribe. It goes without saying that this area should have provision against inclement weather, for exposure to extreme cold is a serious enemy to shock victims, particularly when priority checks may require that some of them be delayed for hours in reaching an area for treatment.

The sorting area must be staffed by personnel who can think and act without dangerous delay. The slogan of "the greatest good for the greatest number" applies here as in few other places. A knowledge of the magnitude of the disaster and if possible some estimate of the number of casualties is essential if the sorting area is to function at its best. Civil defense or some other agency should provide adequate communications promptly.

The doctors in this area must have some idea of how many seriously injured people can be handled in a given period of time and make their decisions accordingly. It is useless for them to give highest priority to a few victims so severely injured that their chances of recovery are almost nil and, in so doing, consume the time of resuscitation and operating personnel, whose efforts might better be devoted to a larger number of critically injured people who have a good chance of survival with prompt therapy. This may seem a heartless approach, but these circumstances require a subordination of certain human emotions that would be praiseworthy under less pressing circumstances.

A diagnosis or at least a clinical classification of each case should be entered on a card securely tied or pinned to the patient's clothing, or better still suspended around his neck, wrist, or ankle. Skin-marking pencils may be used in some cases, particularly to denote narcotics and tetanus inoculations given, provided there is a clear understanding of any code used.

The patients should be moved out of the sorting area through a preplanned chain of evacuation to various areas or departments of the hosiptal where their course will be followed by further observation, emergency treatment, and definitive treatment. Little definitive treatment is justified in large disasters if it endangers the lives of other waiting patients. Pride in accurate reduction of fractures and neat closure of wounds must give way to an assembly line production that keeps the channels open and the traffic moving. The physicians must think in terms of survival and not cosmetic results. The things necessary to prevent further shock or hemorrhage must be known and applied and more definitive efforts aimed at perfect end results postponed until a more optimum time.

The areas in which a given type of study or treatment is carried out may not be the ones used for that purpose, under standard operating practice. Obviously, the x-ray department remains the x-ray department, but the nurses' dining room may become a shock or resuscitation ward, and the physical therapy department may be turned into a minor surgical or fracture department.

The type of injuries resulting from a disaster will dictate the amount of activity in the various departments, but thinking and planning must be elastic to provide for any eventuality. Probably any hospital disaster plan should provide burn, shock, and fracture areas, a "minor surgery" area (much as I dislike that term), and a preoperative preparation area. None of these can be clear-cut as to function and activity, for a patient may be burned, have a fractured femur, and be in shock. Obviously, such a patient is in a serious condition and should be cared for in an area where the personnel will recognize his danger and take immediate steps to prevent his condition from worsening. Definitive treatment of the femur should be postponed, but it must be well splinted to remove one of the underlying causes of shock. The shock must be treated first, and even if the patient doesn't show signs of shock but his femur is fractured and he is severely burned, he is a candidate for shock and should be treated accordingly. A most important virtue of the good emergency department doctor is his ability to recognize potential shock.

Space Is Needed for Burn Care

The area of the hospital indicated for the care of burns should, if possible, be one or more large rooms. Many small private rooms or treatment rooms are not satisfactory as they require more personnel for close observation of these patients.

The causes of death from burns should be kept in mind and necessary equipment to combat these provided. Among these is obstruction to the airway. This may occur from burns of the face and neck, as edema causes obstruction. Tracheostomy sets must be in readiness for this. In severe face and neck burns, prophylactic tracheostomy is often advisable as it is much easier to do before edema of the neck occurs. This not only relieves obstruction but provides easy access for aspiration of secretions. These are often profuse, particularly when fumes or steam have been inhaled so that they irritate the trachea and bronchi. Care of the tracheostomy is important as a patient may choke to death from his own secretions below the level of the tracheostomy. Aspiration is a simple procedure, not difficult to teach to any attendant, but it is well to begin the instruction before the emergency arises. The irritants inhaled in burns of the respiratory tract may cause pulmonary edema and, if there is evidence of this, fluids must be given with caution.

Burn Shock

Extensive deep burns destroy large numbers of red blood cells by direct heat and also increase the fragility of these cells so that hemolysis may occur. It has been estimated that more than 25 percent of the circulating red cells may be destroyed in extensive burns. Damage is also done to the surface capillaries, resulting in loss of fluid from the circulation. The vasodilation and increased capillary permeability resulting from burns also reduces the circulating blood volume, and in turn hypoxia of the tissues occurs. The standard measures for treating reduced blood volume must be available in the burn area and must include the plasma volume expanders but, particularly, solutions for the replacement of lost electrolytes. Lactated Ringer's solution is a valuable one here. If burns are not deep, there is not much need for whole blood, for there is little red cell destruction; but in full thickness burns, there is great red cell destruction, and whole blood must be available.

A working liaison with the laboratory is of course necessary for cross matching and for hematocrit readings.

Train Others to Give Oxygen

In dealing with the causes of death from burns, that is, respiratory obstruction and shock, oxygen is of extreme importance, and it must be available so that it can be given promptly. Here again, the predisaster training of personnel is important. There will not be enough anesthetists, doctors, or even nurses to administer oxygen in some cases. Other personnel must be taught, even if they do not know the reasons back of what they are doing.

In addition to facilities to combat death from burns, other preparations must be made in the burn area to prevent infection and to guard against delayed shock. Wound cleansing, as in any open wound, will help prevent infection. It must be remembered that heat is a great sterilizer and that many of these burned surfaces have been thus sterilized. Contamination must not be added to an otherwise fairly clean surface. Attendants should wear caps and masks just as they would in an operating room. Extensive debridement should not be done, but loose burned tissue and dirt should be removed. This may be done with forceps, scissors, and by sponging or irrigating with sterile saline.

General anesthesia is not advisable in burned patients and is seldom needed. Pain may be controlled by intravenous narcotics.

Care of burns following the initial cleansing may depend on the experience of the involved physicians. I believe that the occlusive dressing method has advantages over the exposure method, particularly when burns cover opposed surfaces of the body. It helps to prevent air contamination, which is a factor in large rooms with many people.

Stockpiling of different sizes of sterile burn dressings in advance of need will save much time. The largest of these should be large enough to cover the entire front or back surface of the trunk or to wrap around an extremity. The surface of the dressing should be fine-mesh gauze or other nonadherent material. I believe small amounts of petrolatum in the gauze help prevent adherence to the burned surface. If time permits, opposed surfaces such as we find in fingers and toes should be protected from each other by dressings. Sterile cotton gloves may be used as hand and finger dressings. As these dressings usually do not require changing for several days, they will, along with any indicated lifesaving measures mentioned above, finish emergency treatment and allow the personnel to proceed with the care of other casualties.

The psychological treatment of the burned patient is most important. Most of these people are frightened, and calm reassurance along with other therapy may be of great value.

Areas for Care of Shock and Fracture Cases

Wound shock has so much in common with burn shock that the area for management of these casualties may well be adjacent to or combined with that for care of burns.

Attempts have been made to eliminate the word "shock" from medical literature. These attempts are ill advised, for if the term is dropped, a great void will remain. There has been much confusion and misinterpretation in the use of this word, but it must be borne in mind that after several decades of redefining and modifying the meaning of the term, it now portrays to the average physician a clinical picture that calls for certain definite action. The cause of shock, in addition to severe burns, may be hemorrhage and damage to body tissue. Pain is a factor, but this is actually a symptom, not really a cause. While a detailed discussion of the mechanism of shock is not germane to these remarks, a brief summary of the sequence of events will point up the treatment required.

Hemorrhage, particularly rapid hemorrhage, or extensive tissue damage, such as broken bones and torn muscles, throws the body into a defensive state which usually starts with vasoconstriction. The circulating blood volume is decreased and the vasoconstriction is a defense against this. This response is due to hypersecretion of the adrenals, which also speeds up the heart. The decreased amount of circulating blood leads to hypoxia, and this in turn interferes with various body functions. Although the blood pressure may be normal or even elevated with the initial vasoconstriction, it will surely drop if the causes of shock are not dealt with. It is because of this that the recognition of the situations that cause shock is of equal importance with the recognition of shock itself. If these are recognized in time, shock may be prevented or at least well controlled. If they are not recognized and the blood pressure drops impressively, a more serious phase of shock which includes an increase in permeability of the capillaries ensues, and the patient's condition becomes more critical.

When I mentioned before the advantage of having nurses who would take and *record* blood pressure readings, I had this in mind. The trend of the blood pressure is just as important as the pressure itself, and if pressures are not recorded, no one can remember what they were, and consequently one of the best guides to the condition of the patient is lost. Hematocrit readings and other laboratory studies are of value, but a laboratory overwhelmed with such requests may not be able to fulfill them. Blood pressure and pulse readings carefully recorded with the time marked are the best practical guides.

There must be some individual in the shock area to whom

is assigned the responsibility of coordinating the activities and keeping a close watch on the progress of patients, in order that a patient not be allowed to go into irreversible shock because no one is watching his progress.

Surgeons interested in care of fractures would naturally be the ones particularly capable in this phase of disaster plan activity and, if plenty of orthopedic and general surgeons are available, this section may be manned by them entirely.

However, some of this personnel may be needed in operating rooms, and other specialists or general practitioners may have to treat fractures. The important thing to remember is that proper splinting will often keep a fracture in position so that it may be reduced at a later time quite satisfactorily. I am not advocating the delayed treatment of fractures under ordinary circumstances, but it has been demonstrated that excellent results can be obtained with definitive reduction done several days after the fracture occurs. Certainly, if these results are to be expected, a knowledge of good splinting methods will help.

There is no better way to hold long-bone fractures of the lower extremities in good position than by application of traction splints. Unfortunately, the traction splint comes in for criticism from time to time, often by physicians who do not understand or even try to understand its value. Their criticism sometimes negates excellent first-aid teaching that well-meaning laymen receive. One of the groups who seem to oppose the Thomas or traction splint is composed of young orthopedic surgeons who look on a fracture as a potential operation and consequently do not care whether the bones are held in good position initially or not. It would be most unfair to say that this includes all young orthopedic surgeons: many of them are advocates of the Thomas splint and know that it will save many fractured bones from surgery. As I never miss an opportunity to praise the traction splint, I have inserted these thoughts here, but other good splints and sterile dressings for use on wounds accompanying the fractures should also be available in the fracture area.

It should be remembered that serious open fractures are surgical emergencies and should have operative treatment if possible, if infection and long convalescence are to be avoided. Such fracture cases should be transferred to the preoperative area to take their place in line for the operating room. Where personnel is available, many fractures may be given definitive treatment by application of casts and thus make possible discharge from the hospital the same day or at an early date.

For Preoperative Care and Lesser Surgery

While all surgery is of major importance, in the situation under discussion some surgical problems may be handled by other than completely trained surgeons, and these cases may well be directed to an area supplied with suture material, dressings, and bandages. Some of these patients may be ambulatory and some may be stretcher cases, but proper cleansing of their wounds and the application of sterile dressings are most important. The distinction between contamination of a wound and infection must be remembered, and thorough wound irrigation and removal of foreign bodies in contaminated wounds may often prevent infection. These steps, along with sterile dressings, are more important than suturing, as secondary suturing is easily done later on a clean wound. Control of bleeding must be carefully done, as hematomas make excellent culture media. The choice between definitive treatment and good first aid on these patients with lesser injuries depends on the time element.

This section of the hospital may best be a ward or wards near the operating room suite. It naturally overlaps in function with the shock area, as some of the patients treated in the latter will be candidates for operation. My concept of a preoperative area is one where patients who need and are ready for surgery are placed. They may be undergoing shock treatment but are showing sufficient improvement to indicate that they are ready, or soon will be, for surgery.

This department needs good surgical judgment and supervision. It is not a good plan to have surgeons come out of the operating room, take a quick look around, and say, "I'll take this one next." It is better to have someone with surgical training observing these patients over a period of time, so that he may know whether they are improving and thus know which patients are most in need of immediate operation.

This may seem to reduce the operating surgeon to the category of a sterile technician, but it is better than having him make snap judgments on a group of patients whom he has not studied.

The surgical personnel working in the operating rooms and in the preoperative area may change places at times and thus be relieved of doing the same type of work over a long period of time.

Other Departments Will Speed Up

Departments which will not be displaced by disaster planning and will function in their normal ways, except at accelerated speed, do not need as much planning, but they do need to shape their thinking to the probable needs.

Laboratory

The physical location of the laboratory will not be changed. However, the use of certain rooms and facilities may be altered in the disaster plan. Most important is the availability of adequate personnel and the assurance that they are imbued with the overall philosophy of concentration on essentials to the exclusion of fancy details. Routine tests on patients already in the hospital should be put aside and preparations made for prompt and accurate support in the care of patients in more critical condition. Blood typing and the availability of adequate amounts of blood deserve serious predisaster planning. Small and medium-sized hospitals cannot be expected to carry in stock in their blood banks sufficient blood for the demands of a major disaster, but arrangements to supplement the available supply from other sources should be made.

X-ray Department

Here again, routine elective work must be pushed aside. There is no time for barium enemas when a line of fresh fracture cases is waiting.

X-ray studies need not be as complete in many cases as they would be under normal circumstances, but they must provide the information needed by the physicians caring for the injured.

Needless to say, supplies in both laboratory and x-ray departments must be available in quantities equal to the heavy demands of many admissions.

Central Supply

As in the blood bank, it would not be feasible in central supply to stockpile everything that might be needed for emergency care of many times the average number of injured patients. There are, however, certain items that should be stocked in excess of routine needs. Foremost among these are burn dressings. These dressings, in several sizes, may be safely kept for long periods of time and resterilized at intervals dictated by experience. The same may be said of other dressings. Instruments for suture trays and for use in the operating rooms may be sterilized by the acceptable methods in use in each hospital, provided personnel is available. Getting the people back on duty to handle the extra work load is what will spell success in this department.

Dietary Department

Food is probably the last thing that a severely injured patient wants. However, as hours pass following his injury, and as he responds to treatment, this desire will return. Special diets in quantity may or may not be called for.

The first problem to be faced by the dietary department is the feeding of extra personnel, doctors who usually eat at home, extra heavy shifts of nurses—in fact, many extra people who normally would not be fed at the hospital but who must be fed in the emergency in order that they may continue to work at peak efficiency. Not only food but the personnel to prepare it outside of regular hours must be planned for. The place where food would ordinarily be served may have to be changed if, for instance, as mentioned before, the nurses' dining room is taken over for the shock ward. While this department may have no direct contact with the injured, it provides one of the basic supports to the whole disaster plan project.

Medical Records

This is one phase of the whole program where details must not be skipped. Records should be accurate and complete. It will be impossible for the normal personnel of the records department to carry this load. There must be supplementary help that is prearranged. This may include extra nurses, if available, secretaries from other departments, volunteers from outside the hospital, or even physicians if some of these are in specialties removed from the skills applicable to the injured. The keeping of good records of the injured is not beneath the dignity of any physician.

Well-prepared and adequately stocked forms are a boon to good records, and the recorders must work with the physicians so that chronological accounts of changing conditions of patients and therapeutic measures used may be recorded in sequence. A physician cannot be expected to remember how a patient looked or what he did to the patient an hour before dictating the record—when, in the meantime, he has cared for others.

Information Center

In any large catastrophe, persons who have no connection with the care of the injured will collect in large numbers. These are not necessarily the idle curious, although they may be. Family and friends of the victims, representatives of the press, the police, and others have a right to know what is going on, yet their presence in the wrong place may interfere with the very procedures which they wish to be successful.

An organized center for the quick, accurate, and courteous dissemination of information must be set up. This may be in the hospital lobby or elsewhere, but it should be far enough away from the point where patients are being admitted to prevent any interference with the care of the injured. This area should be well marked, and police and others should direct the public to it for information.

This center may be staffed by Red Cross workers or others who will get and keep information about the victims so that it may be given out. Contact between this center and the treatment area is important. Some reporters will not be satisfied with this arrangement. They will want to sneak through a corridor and get a first-hand story in the emergency department. Someone in authority, even the police if necessary, should prevent this. Nothing could be worse than to have an inexperienced layman witnessing and interpreting to the public things he doesn't understand. When those in charge of the care of patients want to let the reporters in, they will, but until then reporters have no business beyond the information center. Needless to say, the handling of this problem requires tact, but above all it requires firmness.

The Clergy

The presence of the clergy in the treatment area is another matter. Most ministers, priests, and rabbis are quite cooperative and will not overstep the bounds. Their presence may be a real help in the care of the severely injured, and within limits they should be allowed to minister to the victims. They are always able to offer comfort to family and friends.

A Cooperative Venture in Keeping Faith

The philosophy of the care of large numbers of casualties as presented here may be distasteful to some, but those who have had the responsibility for dealing with such situations will not find it so. We all like to do work of which we are proud, and we dislike a second-best effort, but the planning for care of mass casualties should consider the overall first-rate effort, not each individual case. If the patient load in a disaster turns out to be lighter than expected, the philosophy as presented here may be toned down and more definitive care given to each patient, but the basic thinking should be predicated on a maximum catastrophe.

A disaster plan in a civilian hospital is a cooperative venture. It is not just a medical staff activity, nor an administrative exercise, nor a facet of the training program for nurses: the plan is all these and more. It is a scheme of action calculated to assure that the hospital will not be found wanting when confronted with a massive emergency for which experience has not prepared it. It requires subordination of personal and selfish desires in the interest of total achievement. A hospital which lacks such a plan or fails to rehearse it periodically is not keeping faith with those who make the institution possible.

When this address was given, the general public was still reacting from World War II. The memory of the destruction wrought by nuclear bombs was still clear. Civil Defense organizations were stressing bomb shelters, but most people had a fatalistic attitude toward this sort of thing. Either they were not interested or they thought it would be of no use for them to become interested. This feeling pervaded the thinking of many hospital people, so it was difficult to arouse enthusiasm about disaster plans. Since that time, there have been a number of civil disasters that have shown hospitals that it does pay to be ready when disaster strikes a community.

The American Medical Association developed a committee on disaster medical care which correlated the experiences of those involved with care of disaster victims. In 1965, this committee published a report based on experiences in five midwestern tornadoes.[3] This report had previously appeared in *Group Practice*, June 1965. Highlights of this report as it relates to hospital emergency services include the following:

1. Standing generators for electricity were sometimes inadequate or unconnected with all needed services, such as x-ray department, switchboard, emergency rooms, and paging mechanisms.

2. In some instances, patients had to be carried up several flights of stairs because electricity was not available to operate the elevators.

3. Many tracheostomies were necessary because of injuries from flying wet mud or head injuries.

4. Warning systems regarding impending disaster were frequently inadequate. This includes warnings to stay out of vehicles and to seek shelter in basements if possible.

5. Critiques of disaster experiences by doctors and others are necessary.

6. Alternate plans for emergency facilities should be considered in case the hospital is damaged by a tornado.

The Committee on Trauma of the American College of Surgeons has also been interested in gaining experience from surveys of the care of the injured in civil disasters. Results of several of these surveys have been published. Two of these involved railroad wrecks in 1962. They were investigated by representatives from the American College of Surgeons. The writer had the opportunity to make one of these surveys, and his report is presented here essentially as it was published in the *Bulletin of the American College of Surgeons.*[4]

REPORT OF A SURVEY OF THE CARE OF THE INJURED IN A PENNSYLVANIA RAILROAD TRAIN WRECK AT STEELTON, PENNSYLVANIA ON JULY 28, 1962

Steelton is a town of 11,000 people lying directly east of Harrisburg and adjoining the main line of the Pennsylvania Railroad on its north side. Steelton has no hospitals, but it may be considered as part of the Greater Harrisburg area so does have quick access to two large, well-equipped and well-staffed general hospitals in Harrisburg. These are the Harrisburg Hospital and the Harrisburg Polyclinic Hospital, each having approximately six hundred beds.

Harrisburg has been the scene of several catastrophes in the past which have resulted in a number of people being killed and injured. The records indicate that one of the worst of these occurred on May 11, 1905, when two passenger trains of the Pennsylvania Railroad plowed into a wrecked freight train which was carrying a car loaded with dynamite. This occurred about two miles west of the July 28, 1962, wreck. Twenty-five people were killed, and one hundred and twenty-five were injured. Horse-drawn vehicles and streetcars were used to transport the injured to the Harrisburg Hospital. Ambulances were not available and neither were stretchers. Shutters were torn from houses by doctors and nurses and used to transport the injured. This wreck occurred near midnight, and hospital personnel worked until noon the next day in the initial care of the injured. A review of more recent history indicates that about ten years ago, there was a wreck of a large bus in which some were killed and many injured. Influenced by these disasters and others and by the general interest across the country in hospital disaster plans, both of the general hospitals in Harrisburg had formulated detailed plans for handling mass casualties.

At the Harrisburg Hospital, the overall plan was broken down into Plans A, B, and C: A to be used in case of twenty to fifty casualties, B in fifty to one hundred, and C when more than one hundred casualties were involved. These three plans centered around a program of the rapid expansion of inpatient facilities, each plan calling for the erection of cots in certain designated areas in accordance with a predetermined pattern. At the Polyclinic Hospital, the outline of the disaster plan was slightly different. It included, first, an *internal disaster*, such as a fire or an explosion, and then three plans depending on the size of the disaster when patients were to be admitted to the hospital. These were classified as *minor emergency*, three to ten casualties; Plan A, ten to forty casualties; and Plan B, over forty casualties. The details under the breakdown here centered more around personnel than expansion of facilities, the latter being expressed in general terms. Each of the three plans, other than the *internal disaster*, specified what hospital personnel was to be utilized and, in the case of the larger disaster, specified aid from outside agencies.

The commendable behavior of personnel at both hospitals indicated that their disaster plans had gone well beyond the paper stage. Saturday evening could be considered a very poor time to expect a favorable response in such an emergency, but such a response was seen at both institutions and demonstrates clearly what may be expected from dedicated personnel working in voluntary hospitals unfettered by regimentation.

The Wreck

At 5:02 P.M. on Saturday, July 28, 1962, a special train headed for the Phillies-Pirate baseball game in Philadelphia left the Harrisburg station two minutes after schedule. There were nine cars drawn by engine number 4878, the largest type in passenger service on the Pennsylvania Railroad. Three minutes later, a smelter foreman in the Bethlehem Steel Company's plant at Steelton, just east of Harrisburg, saw the train as it was rapidly gaining full speed on the straight stretch of level four-track road bed that passes between the open-hearth furnaces and the Susquehanna River. As he reflected on the fact that he had refused permission to his fifteen-year-old son to make this trip to the night game in Philadelphia, he was horrified to see the last four coaches begin to bounce as they left the tracks and then saw the last three disappear out of sight as they rolled down the thirty-foot bank into the river on the other side of the tracks. He notified the steel company office, and the record in the office of the Chief of Police in Steelton shows that they were notified of the wreck and its location at 5:15 P.M. This call came from a guard at the Bethlehem Steel plant. The police log also indicates that they immediately sent officers in cruise cars to the scene of the accident and notified the township police, Harrisburg police, the two ambulance squads in Steelton, fire companies, American Red Cross Headquarters, and Dauphin County Civil Defense. The Civil Defense Headquarters in turn alerted all ambulance squads in the area. The telephone operator at the Harrisburg Hospital reports that, at 5:23 P.M., she received a call from the Bethlehem Steel Company's plant alerting the hospital about the wreck. The medical director of the hospital, who is usually not in his office at this time on Saturday, had returned to the hospital to get some papers which he wanted to work on over the weekend. He was notified of the situation and boarded an ambulance along with two interns and a driver and left immediately for the scene of the accident, arriving about 5:40 P.M. After an initial estimate of the situation and immediate advice to those who had preceded him, he went back to a telephone in the Bethlehem Steel plant, over two hundred yards away, to call the hospital. He then immediately returned to aid in the care of the injured and in the evacuation of the casualties. His driver had been unable to get the ambulance closer than about three hundred yards to the scene of the wreck due to certain physical obstructions, such as railroad tracks within the grounds of the steel plant. This prevented use of the ambulance radio for easy communication with the hospital. From then on, the medical director's only contact with the hospital was by sending messages with the ambulance drivers as they returned to the hospital. No portable radios or mobile telephones were available at that time. When the medical director arrived, many people were industriously caring for the injured, but no one was in charge and the efforts were not organized. Being well known in the community, he was recognized as a physician and, with the help of several other physicians from the community, he was able to get some order to the care of the injured. The first casualty arrived at the Harrisburg Hospital by ambulance at about 6:00 P.M. The medical director returned there a little after 7:00 P.M.

Difficulties in Rescue and Evacuation

Several circumstances and the physical layout at the scene of the wreck made the care and evacuation of the injured unusually difficult. Four poles with high tension wires carrying 132,000 volts of current were knocked down, leaving the wires across the tracks. Until this current was cut off, this presented a very dangerous hazard to rescue operations. Several children who crawled out of the wrecked cars were warned by railroad personnel to stay off the tracks and away from the wires. The live wires had set fire to grass and brush between the railroad tracks and the steel plant, and the wounded had to be carried across this field to the ambulances. The cars were partially submerged in the water, adding to the difficulty of gaining an entrance to them, and the injured had to be carried up a steep bank and across the tracks to level ground and then nearly three hundred yards to the waiting ambulances. Lack of overall control by a law enforcement officer in the early stages of the rescue reduced the efficiency of the willing, eager, and capable participants in the rescue. One interesting and rather fantastic incident in this connection concerned the hijacking of an ambulance. A woman who had had a very severe injury to her arm but who was not in critical condition as far as life was concerned had been loaded on an ambulance but, because the driver was not immediately available, the woman's husband, who had been slightly injured in the wreck, jumped into the

driver's seat and took off with the ambulance on his own authority, taking his wife to the Polyclinic Hospital. It was
reported that the driver of this ambulance, finding his ambulance gone and the other Polyclinic Hospital ambulances waiting, drove it to the hospital, leaving the proper driver of the
second ambulance without a vehicle. Thus, two ambulance
drivers temporarily lost their vehicles due to the lack of organized dispatching.

Many Volunteers

The prompt and willing response of many agencies and many
individuals in the handling of this disaster was most pleasing.
Any criticism that might be directed at the efforts could certainly not be leveled at those who responded, but rather at a
certain lack of coordination. Among those who came to the
scene and participated in the rescue and evacuation of the
wounded were the city and state police, all area rescue units
which provided thirty ambulances, the local Civil Defense
organization, the American Red Cross, a helicopter crew
from the Middletown Air Force Base, the telephone company,
and personnel from both general hospitals. Some ambulances
came from twenty to thirty miles away, and a Red Cross team
came from twenty miles away and helped with first aid at the
scene of the accident. The personnel of this team stayed until
3:00 a.m. in order to provide first aid for any individuals injured in the process of clearing up the wreck after the wounded
from the wreck had been removed. The Bethlehem Steel Company police also participated in the rescue work, and it was
reported that fifty fire companies in the area were alerted, and
many responded to aid with the rescue. A firemen's parade in a
nearby town was halted, and many of these firemen went directly to the scene. The Steelton police notified the River Rescue
Squad, and they responded with boats and trained crews. Particular mention should be made of the Bainbridge Naval
Station drill team. This group of young sailors was passing
nearby and went to the scene of the rescue and did an excellent job in getting people out of the cars. Six minutes after the

Air Force base had been notified, a helicopter was airborne. It flew over the wreck and then landed one hundred yards away. Two injured were evacuated by this helicopter to the Harrisburg Hospital; one was dead on arrival, but the other was admitted for treatment. The helicopter landed on a grass-covered area by the river bank in front of the Harrisburg Hospital.

Traffic Control

According to reports, traffic control was superior. All auxiliary police of the Steelton Police Force were called out, and the main street leading from in front of the steel plant toward Harrisburg was freed of unnecessary traffic. An officer was placed at each intersection, and he prevented entrance onto this street of any vehicles not connected with the evacuation of the injured. Good traffic control also prevailed in the city of Harrisburg, and there was little interference with the passage of the ambulances from the scene of the wreck to the two Harrisburg hospitals.

The Dead

Many of the deaths in this wreck were violent ones. Bodies were dismembered and, in one case, a child was decapitated. Death was probably instant in practically all cases. I was able to obtain only one report of an instance where an individual was still breathing although obviously lethally injured. This was a woman whose leg had been amputated and who had also sustained an abdominal evisceration. She was apparently still breathing when the rescue efforts started but died very promptly after this. The bodies, many of which were removed from the cars with great difficulty, were brought out, placed on stretchers, and taken to a temporary morgue in the Bethlehem Steel plant. A large rectangular building with a concrete floor was designated for this purpose, and it is unfortunate that the bodies were not left there until they were removed to mortuaries. The coroner ordered the bodies removed to the morgue at the Polyclinic Hospital, and 16 of the 19 dead were taken there. This, of course, added to the administrative load at the Polyclinic Hospital, and the presence of family and friends identifying the dead produced some confusion.

The Injured

The newspaper report on Sunday morning following the accident stated that there had been 140 passengers and crew on the train and that, of these, nineteen had been killed and one hundred injured. It is obvious that this estimate of the number injured was low. Officials at the Harrisburg Hospital state that over one hundred were treated there and twenty-five admitted. The Polyclinic Hospital record indicates that, in addition to the sixteen dead being brought there, ten were treated for injuries and seven admitted. Of the twenty-five patients admitted to the Harrisburg Hospital, eleven were reported to have had fractures, and of the seven at the Polyclinic Hospital, four to have had fractures. One of the fracture patients at the Harrisburg Hospital had an open fracture of the shaft of the femur, and two had compression fractures of the spine. A witness reported that most of the severe fractures were in the dead. Three days after the wreck, twenty-one of the twenty-five admitted patients remained in the Harrisburg Hospital, and six of the seven in the Polyclinic Hospital. Of these twenty-seven patients, two were reported as serious, eight as unsatisfactory, and seventeen as satisfactory. At the time of this survey, two weeks after the wreck, seventeen of the patients remained in the two hospitals.

Hospital Preparations

Sixty members of the medical staff reported at the Harrisburg Hospital within one and one-half hours after the accident and a similar number at the Polyclinic Hospital. The majority of these were surgeons and orthopedists. Other necessary personnel as stipulated in the disaster plans of the hospital was called. The administrator of the Harrisburg Hospital reported that practically all key people from the hospital responded to the call promptly. A similar report came from the Polyclinic Hospital where, as events developed, there was a considerable surplus of medical personnel. The chief technician of the Harrisburg Hospital blood bank put out a radio call for blood donors, requesting particularly "O" positive and "O" negative blood. Thirty minutes after this call, sixty volunteers had shown up, and before long, one hundred had come in. The Pennsylvania Society of Medical Technologists and Laboratory Technicians was having a meeting at the Harrisburg Hospital, and the members volunteered for work in drawing blood. Thirty-two donors were bled that evening and ten pints of blood were given. Fifteen were given later to wreck victims. The Harrisburg Hospital usually carries about two hundred pints of blood in the bank, but they were particularly concerned about the shortage of "O" negative. They communicated with the Polyclinic Hospital, where there were fewer injured sent, and were assured that they could help supplement the blood supply if necessary. At the Harrisburg Hospital, preconceived planning resulted in rapid expansion of the emergency facilities. The seriously injured stretcher cases were brought into the emergency room proper, which is adequate in size for a hospital of this type. The less seriously injured walking wounded were sent to the fourth floor in the clinic area; a third area was designated where those who had been treated and needed to be detained for observation or who were waiting for x-ray reports were sent. Thus, the emergency room proper, where the more seriously injured were being given immediate treatment, was not cluttered up with less seriously injured people. Thirty cots were set up and made ready in the gymnasium of the nurses' home, which communicates with the hospital with an underground tunnel. Sixteen nurses were assigned there and not allowed to leave. Twenty more cots were in readiness to be set up in the gymnasium if needed. At the Polyclinic Hospital, where there is a quite modern emergency department that would take care of any usual group of patients from automobile accidents and so forth, the facilities were also immediately expanded. A large rectangular clinic waiting room which is close to the emergency department was emptied of chairs and prepared for the reception of stretcher cases. At the Harrisburg Hospital where most of the wounded were being treated and admitted, plans were put into effect to prevent cluttering up the emergency department with friends, relatives, press, and so forth. An information center was set up in the hospital lobby and the "gray ladies" of the American Red Cross were of great assistance here. Lists of the names of those injured were brought out to this information center as quickly as possible, and supplementary lists including the addresses and later the injuries of the patients were added at intervals. An attempt was made to keep the press out of the emergency room and to give information to reporters at the information center. Long-distance calls came in from as far away as Toronto, Ontario, asking for details on the wreck, and these were handled from the information center. Before midnight, a complete list of all injured who had been brought to the hospital, along with their addresses and types of injuries, had been completed. The hospital authorities report that, by 11:00 p.m., all the injured had been cared for, emergency surgery had been done, and the soot, blood, cinders, and so forth were being cleaned up in the emergency department. The administrators of both hospitals, who are laymen, both stated repeatedly how pleased they were with the attitude of everyone in this emergency. The administrator at the Harrisburg Hospital stated that no one questioned his job and that no one felt that his assignment was beneath him even though, in one case, several physicians were assigned only to keep records which they made by typewriter. It is interesting to note that the Harrisburg Hospital, which is in a downtown area, is usually fairly busy in its emergency department on Saturday evening and that all of the routine emergency cases and casual visitors to this department were taken care of in addition to those brought from the wreck. At the Polyclinic Hospital, where the activities were less concentrated, press relations and information was handled through the information center in the medical library as designated in their disaster plan. Tagging of patients with name, address, diagnosis, and so forth was done at the hospitals as the patients were brought in. I was unable to get very definite information with regard to two phases of the emergency care. No one seemed to be very clear as to how the long-bone fractures had been splinted. I was informed that some of the ambulances were supplied with traction splints and others with various other types of splints. I have the impression from speaking to some of the physicians, including the chief surgeon of the Bethlehem Steel Company, that some of the fractured patients may have been transported without splinting. Information with regard to tetanus immunization was also sketchy, and I am unable to make an accurate statement as to how this was handled.

It should be stated that at the Polyclinic Hospital, although no wounded were evacuated there by helicopter, preparations had been made for this type of transportation. A vacant lot across the street from the hospital had been cleared of cars and the ground sprayed with chemicals such as are used at air strips when emergency landings are to be made, that is, chemicals to prevent the outbreak of fire.

Summary

The preceding description of events connected with this Pennsylvania Railroad wreck, and the handling of the injured following it, is based on the observations made by an outside and unbiased observer in a two-day study two weeks after the wreck. This study consisted of conferences with many people who were involved in the handling of this disaster, as well as a careful inspection of the scene of the accident, the ambulance routes between it and the hospitals, and of the facilities in the hospitals themselves. As far as the hospitals are concerned, it is difficult to do anything but praise the efforts of the personnel there. At both institutions, the effects of predisaster planning were evident. Much praise is also due to many other agencies in the community and to many individuals. Any shortcomings that appear as a result of the care of this disaster are ones of lack of coordination rather than lack of willingness and ability on the part of people concerned. The shortcomings that I will point out are not based entirely on my own opinion, but are listed after careful consideration based on discussions with those who were involved and who themselves were eager to find their own mistakes. Weaknesses in the handling of the injured of this wreck come to light in four areas:

1. *At the scene.* Although there were many volunteers, both among amateurs and professionals who participated in the rescue efforts, there does seem to have been a lack of overall direction to their efforts, particularly in the time immediately following the accident. As time progressed, natural leaders developed and abilities were recognized and those who needed guidance turned to these for help, but the overall command by a law enforcement officer who would use as his lieutenants those with various skills and abilities would have hastened and improved the completion of the job.

2. *Transportation.* Hindsight would suggest that the quick procurement of some planks which could have been piled on either side of the rails of the tracks that the ambulances did not want to drive over, would have allowed the ambulances to come within one hundred to one hundred and fifty feet of the injured people rather than to have to stop three hundred yards away. This would have shortened the litter carry and would have brought the ambulance radios into usable distance by physicians at the scene of the accident who could have notified the hospitals as to just what to expect. As it was, the hospitals were in the dark, having no idea as to approximately how many injured or what types of injured would be coming to them. A more effective dispatching of the ambulances would also have been of great value. Where large numbers of injured have to be evacuated, particularly if they are going to more than one hospital, a central dispatching agency or authority will better distribute the injured to the facilities prepared, thus relieving an overload at one point and giving the willing workers at another place more to do.

3. *Communications.* For a considerable period of time after the wreck, there was complete lack of communications between the scene of the accident and hospitals and other cooperating areas. I am told that the local Civil Defense has portable radios. If these walkie-talkies had been brought immediately to the scene of the accident, it would have been of great help to the medical director of the Harrisburg Hospital, who had no

way to send messages back to his hospital except by word of mouth to ambulance drivers. It is reported that portable telephones were installed later, but the reports that I received were that this was done after all of the injured had been removed and, consequently, after the time that they were most direly needed.

4. *Disposition of the dead.* It was a big mistake to take the dead to the Polyclinic Hospital. If this hospital had had the same patient load that the Harrisburg Hospital had, it would have resulted in the tying up of needed professional personnel and would have added to the confusion. It would be much better to leave the bodies in the temporary morgue until they could be transported to mortuaries.

Final note: The survey of this wreck was very interesting and instructive to me, and I believe that it was instructive to many of the people who cooperated with me. I was most fortunate to be in Harrisburg on the evening when one hour of television time was devoted to a summary of the care of the injured in this wreck. Many of those who had participated in the care of the injured, as well as those who had furnished other services in this connection, appeared on television and told their story. I was invited to participate in the program to give the impressions obtained by my survey as well as to offer constructive criticism. I was given four or five minutes of television time and quickly summarized the high points of the above report.

I had been able, before going to Harrisburg, to make some preparation for this survey by writing to several interested people. I had corresponded with Doctor William McBride, the Chief of Surgery at Polyclinic Hospital; and with Doctor Champe C. Pool, Orthopedic Surgeon at Polyclinic Hospital and Chairman of the Regional Trauma Committee of the American College of Surgeons; and with Doctor W. Paul Dailey, Medical Director, Harrisburg Hospital. They had been helpful in alerting others who might be able to help with this survey. Others with whom I conferred were the following:

James R. Doran, Editor, *Harrisburg Patriot News.*
Walter S. Shakespeare, Administrator, Harrisburg Hospital.
Doctor Paul K. Waltz, Chief Surgeon, Steelton Plant, Bethlehem Steel Company.

Doctor R. Edward Steele, Surgeon at Harrisburg Hospital and mem-
    ber, Regional Trauma Committee, American College of Sur-
    geons.
An orthopedic surgeon at the Harrisburg Hospital.
The chief of staff at the Harrisburg Hospital.
Mrs. Roberta Heiden, Chief Technician, Blood Bank, Harrisburg
    Hospital.
The head nurse in the emergency department at the Harrisburg
    Hospital.
J. Lincoln MacFarland, Administrator, Polyclinic Hospital.
Doctor William Bates, Director of Medical Education at the Poly-
    clinic Hospital.
Chief of Police, Steelton, Pennsylvania.
The Disaster Director, American Red Cross.
A major, United States Air Force, who commanded the detachment
    of two helicopters flown to the scene of the accident.
Major General Albert Stackpole, Ret., owner of TV station *WHP* at
    Harrisburg.
A representative from the Pennsylvania Railroad.
A member of the Bethlehem Steel Company's Safety Division who
    was on duty at the time of the wreck.

All of these people, plus others, were most helpful and cooperative in supplying information concerning the wreck and the
care of the injured. I found that, as time went on, I obtained
information from some of these people that either corroborated
or corrected information that I obtained from others. Several
were grateful to have erroneous impressions corrected.

I am convinced that, if a major disaster were to occur again
in the Harrisburg area, this fine cooperative group of community leaders would again do a superior job and that they would
profit by the mistakes which they themselves were able to see.

REFERENCES

1. Amspacher, W.H.: The Role of the Civilian Physician in a Mass Casualty
    Situation. An address presented at Fort Sam Houston, Texas, Mar.
    26, 1963.
2. Spencer, J.H.: Mass casualties in the civilian hospital. *Bull Am Coll
    Surgeons,* 1963.
3. Disaster medical care, *AMA, 1:4,* pp. 5–6.
4. Kennedy, R.H., and Spencer, J.H.: Disaster in Missoula (Kennedy) and
    in Steelton (Spencer). *Bull Am Coll Surgeons,* 47:350–355, 365–371,
    1962.

Chapter 12

COSTS AND FEES

Not all administrators and trustees agree on basic fiscal policies of a hospital. There are some who are interested mainly in the overall balance sheet, hoping that month-by-month income will equal outgo. There are others who interest themselves in the financial success, or lack of it, in each department. Their interest may be largely academic or it may be with the thought in mind that certain departments need to revise their rates or review their expenditures in order to balance the departmental budget. This is not the place to present the pros and cons of having one department support another. Discussions between representatives of hospitals and the Blue Cross bring all the arguments out into the open from time to time, and they are frequently published.

Regardless of the attitude toward distribution of charges and expenses as they relate to inpatients, the emergency department presents a situation that must be dealt with separately. Emergency room supplies as well as employees will of course, come under the overall hospital budget as well as the departmental budget, and it will not be difficult for a hospital accountant to estimate what it costs to operate the department. The matter of revenue from the department can also be reported separately from other hospital income.

Major income-producing departments which show a substantial profit are in some hospitals exploited to balance out deficits in other departments. Where this practice is followed, management risks the ire of those responsible for the profit-producing departments. These people may well argue that their surplus should go into more equipment, more personnel, and improvement in employee benefits rather than be used to "bail out" departments where income does not meet budget. This book is concerned with effectiveness of the emergency department, so an attempt to advise fiscal policy will not be made. It can be said, however, that many emergency departments are self-financing, so it can be done.

With at least tentative estimates in mind, a policy with regard to support of this department must be established. Unless the trustees and the administrator decide to operate the department at a loss as a community service, there is no reason why the rate structure cannot be set up in such a way as to prevent or at least minimize loss. The type of community and thus the type of patient will of course influence results, but if collections are as good as one might expect in this day of "the affluent society," in most communities reasonable emergency rates should result in a balanced departmental budget. An emergency department in a poverty area will not pay expenses, regardless of booked charges, but for that matter the entire hospital may not. Outside subsidy will be needed. In the average community, with a good employment situation, the emergency department can be made to pay its way. Whether management desires this will influence the scale of charges.

The above discussion has to do with cost of and charges for hospital services. The charge for professional services is another matter and has been more than alluded to in the chapter on staffing. The hospital is surely justified in establishing a basic charge for each patient. Occasionally someone will object to this because "nothing was done," but this again will teach patients that if they come to the hospital for medical attention and get it, they must expect a charge, even if there is no "laying on of hands." How much service will be included in the basic charge must be determined, and it is well to recognize that at times someone will have to make a decision regarding added charges. Let us take an example. A child is brought in after falling off her bicycle and cutting her forehead. While the doctor is on the way or finishing up the treatment of the previous patient, a nurse puts the child on a stretcher and amid protests and very little support from the mother, washes the forehead with sterile water and pHisoHex® or some other liquid soap. Up to this point, these services might be expected to be covered by the basic charge of four, five, or six dollars or whatever had been determined as the flat fee. The doctor arrives and instructs the nurse to unwrap a wound irrigation tray and a small suture tray. By the time the treatment is completed, 30 to 40 minutes of the nurse's time have been used, as well as two trays of equipment, including one or two tubes of fine silk, a pair of sterile gloves, and certain dressing materials. If someone were to estimate the time needed to wash the instruments, set up and resterilize the trays, wash and resterilize the gloves, and add this to the cost of the sutures, gauze, bandages, and nurse's salary, it would be quite evident that the basic charge would not cover expenses, without any mention of overhead. This matter is further discussed in Chapter 6 on supplies.

These facts necessitate some kind of scale based on realistic costs, with a certain flexibility in rates that will allow for adjustment by the nurse or other person in charge of the business activities in the department. If the basic charge is as much as Abbott[1] reports it to be in his hospital, that is $6.00 (it has been increased since his report), it may include more than in departments where the charge is kept at a minimum. This charge should be clearly stated to the patient as a hospital charge, to prevent its being confused with the professional charge made by the physician. A receipt should be issued if the bill is paid at the time the service is rendered. On such receipts, some hospitals print or rubber-stamp a statement to the effect that the doctor's charges are not included in this bill. This tends to prevent misunderstandings and makes it easier for the physician to collect the fee due him, either on the spot or by future billing.

These details with regard to costs, billing, and collections can prove quite important particularly in dealing with transient patients. Some such patients may come from communities where they are in the habit of getting much free service from municipal hospitals. It requires a little tact and clear-cut business methods to have them understand that such free services are not available to all comers in all communities. These are "changing times" in which we live and work. The percentage of patients who are not able to pay a fair charge for medical or surgical services has diminished. The fact that some communities and some hospitals have not adjusted their philosophies to these changes is not a valid reason why other communities and other hospitals should suffer when people from the first communities are traveling, visiting, or vacationing.

Elsewhere in this book, the author has made it clear that members of his profession should continue, as traditionally they always have, to provide essential and prompt care to those in need, regardless of their ability to pay. In emergencies the care should come first. However, the fact that the treatment was made necessary because of an emergency does not decrease its intrinsic value or the responsibility of the recipient to pay for it if possible. The time may come when all these things are free, but we have not yet reached that stage. Current planning should be on the pay-as-we-go basis. Hospitals, to a certain extent, are blessed or burdened with some of the same responsibilities carried by the medical profession. Even though they are businesses, they are also professional institutions with a moral obligation to provide care for the sick and injured. The occasional newspaper story recounting an instance of an acutely ill or badly injured patient being refused admission to a hospital, without even an examination, on the basis of inability to pay, leaves a very bad impression on the public. Fortunately, these occurrences are rare. The reference of medically indigent patients not in need of immediate attention to tax-supported hospitals is, of course, another matter.

Responsible as hospitals are to provide prompt service when needed, this in no way relieves those who receive the service from financial responsibility. Exactly the same principle applies as in the case of the physician. The hospital is quite justified in protecting its interests by any reasonable measures. Where the patient is medically indigent, there might well be some give-and-take arrangement by which the municipality that would be responsible if the patient were at home would display the same degree of responsibility when the patient was hospitalized away from home because of an emergency. Government officials purporting to have a deep interest in the medical welfare of the citizenry might give this matter some thought.

While good medical care should always have the highest priority, there is no reason why the business side of the transaction should not be given early attention. Just when the subject of payment should be brought up will be a matter for the nurse to decide or, in a large department, the clerk or secretary. The subject may often be tactfully introduced by such a question as, "You probably have insurance, don't you?" or, "Are you covered by Blue Cross and Blue Shield?" Blue Cross and Blue Shield are so widely known now that nearly everyone understands such a question even if he is not so insured. Introducing the subject of payment by a question about insurance is more tactful than saying, "Do you want to pay for this now?" or some other direct approach, and the next move is then up to the patient or his family. While Blue Cross payments in most cases are made directly to the hospital and Blue Shield payments directly to the doctor, the benefits from many commercial policies are not. It is well to explain this to the patient with the statement that he will be given a receipt for his payment which he may submit to his insurance carrier for reimbursement. While some people know exactly how they are covered, others are quite vague about it. This type of patient may be trying to evade the issue with the hope that he can get out of town with his wounds repaired but his finances intact. Out-of-town patients usually need closer watching than local residents, particularly local people known to the hospital. It will not be time wasted to give nurses and others carrying emergency room responsibilities some basic instruction in the business side of the department.

Much time and trouble may be avoided by keeping in the department report forms for Blue Cross and Blue Shield plans covering people in the area. If the hospital is near a state line where from time to time policy holders from another area are treated, forms from the Blue Cross and Blue Shield associations in those areas should be stocked. The same holds true with regard to forms from commercial insurance carriers writing coverage in the community. This has already been alluded to in Chapter 10 on medical records. The completion of insurance forms before patients leave the emergency department, unless they are to be admitted to the hospital, in a wise and timesaving precaution. It will save much trouble later, and few patients will object. In fact, if the coverage is through the Blue plans, patients will welcome the opportunity to fulfill their entire responsibility on the spot. It should be mentioned that, both in the case of Blue Cross and Blue Shield, there are still a few associations with completely unrealistic fee schedules. Care must be taken not to assure any patient that he will owe nothing in addition to the insurance payments.

Where the patient's total bill involves charges from the laboratory or x-ray departments, care must be taken to get these charges properly included. It is surprising how quickly a bill can add up to a formidable sum after what may not be a very severe injury. Physicians attending patients here must, of course, order any tests really necessary to determine the diagnosis and course of treatment, but some restraint should be exercised. Young doctors, recently out of residency training, may particularly need to be cautioned about this. Skull x-rays are often needlessly ordered. One of the vacuums in some of our best training programs is instruction in what needs to be done and what is only of interest. The order sheet on the average patient on a teaching service in a university hospital would not represent a pattern to be followed in the care of private patients of modest income in a community hospital. Young doctors using it as a pattern should be warned that they may price themselves and their hospital out of the market.

In summary it may be said that:

Emergency department charges should be realistic.

They should be collected on the spot if possible.

An explanation of charges should be given, particularly if requested.

Insurance forms should be completely and promptly filled out.

Useless and unnecessary services should be avoided, in order to keep charges at a minimum.

It should be made clear to the patient that the charge for hospital services does not include the professional charges, unless there is some salaried arrangement with physicians with an understanding that the hospital collects for all services.

The matter of physicians' income from work in the emergency department has been discussed in the chapter on staffing. The decision as to how the professional coverage of the department is to be provided will, of course, include the economic aspect. Fee for services collected by the doctor is the most frequent arrangement in departments where a professional charge is made. The other arrangements, including billing by the hospital (either in the name of the doctor or as part of an all-inclusive fee), or salaries, or hourly payments, have been outlined. Unless the department is operated as a community service with an attempt made to limit the service to the medically indigent, care should be taken not to downgrade the value of good medical attention by bargain basement prices. The interests of members of the medical staff as well as other physicians in the community should be protected. Much of the minor emergency work done in the departments may be done in the doctor's office if the doctors are available and there is a strong probability that it may be done there at less cost. The last thing any hospital should do is enter into competition with the doctors who support it. One of the foundation stones of sound public relations of a hospital is the constant and enthusiastic praise of the hospital by the doctors.

An occasional hospital provides emergency room care at no direct cost to the patient. In some instances, this cost is partially or completely reimbursed by the municipality in various ways. Unless reimbursement is obtained, it must not be forgotten that the costs must be charged off somewhere. This may result in a hidden surcharge to private patients. The practical as well as moral aspect of this should be considered before a policy of free service is established. The author would like to put on record his feeling toward the moral aspect of hidden charges. He has heard hospital people use such expressions as, "Oh well, Blue Cross will pick that up." It is just as wrong to include unrelated expenses in charges to Blue Cross as in charges to an individual. Blue Cross programs are under constant pressure to increase their benefits, yet they often have difficulty in getting approval for premium increases to cover these. The least hospitals can do is not pass over to them costs that are not connected to the service Blue Cross is providing for its policy holders. Of course, in the

former is economically as well as administratively impractical and the latter impossible.

Rusk[1] called attention to the almost insurmountable obstacles that hospitals would have to hurdle to make effective the Medicare program from the standpoint of personnel. This problem we have. It has been created by law. There is no law making it mandatory to provide the type of service the public appears to want in emergency departments. Thought must be given to where this will end or to whether it will end.

In the decision to take a firm stand and give the public what it *needs*, not what it apparently *wants*, requires courage. Those who lack the courage will raise the white flag of public relations and let bad enough alone to get worse. Those who have the courage will face the issue squarely, take all parties into their confidence, and set out to build *sound* public relations. This may vary from what is superficially called "good" public relations. This is what was meant by studying the subject in depth.

If the hospital is a new one or if an emergency department is being constructed for the first time, the task will be simpler. Where it involves a change in policy in a community where bad habits have already developed, it will not be so simple.

In Chapter 1, the campaign instituted by the Ingalls Memorial Hospital, Harvey, Illinois, is described. Such a campaign may be considered in other communities, but the pattern of any such campaign must fit the local needs. Care should be taken in the planning to obtain the opinions of many. There should be general agreement regarding steps to be taken, although unanimous opinion may not be possible. Tact will be required. If there are one or two dissenters who either oppose the idea in principle or feel that it will fail, an attempt should be made to get them at least to remain silent and not try to sabotage the effort.

Whatever the overall plan with regard to the type of service offered to the public in an emergency department, every effort should be made to deal with the public with reason and consideration. People coming to the emergency department are often strangers to the hospital; this is their first contact. They may be suspicious; they are frequently frightened and distraught. More than the usual amount of patience may be called for.

Nothing should be done or said to give the impression that their needs are not taken seriously. Not all doctors, nurses, and others are endowed with equal amounts of human understanding and compassion, but the traits can be developed and should be. Unnecessary delays should be avoided; necessary delays should be explained and everything possible done to give the impression that something is being done. Even moving a patient from the waiting room to the area where he is to be examined and treated will help. With all this in mind, proper priorities should be established. It may be necessary, even in the middle of an examination of a nonemergent patient, to stop and give attention to a later arrival needing and thus deserving prompt attention. Every effort should be made to explain this to the nonemergency patient. This is a splendid opportunity to demonstrate the real function of the department. The waiting patient will know, if he is reasonable, that if he comes to the department with a real emergency, he will be promptly treated.

Any organization dealing with the public may from time to time find it necessary to change certain policies. This need not have an adverse effect on public relations if sound reasons for the changes are presented. The public must be informed through all available media, such as newspapers, radio, Parent-Teacher Associations, service clubs, and even the public schools. Public opinion is molded by these and will be molded on the basis of available information. Not only should the trustees of a hospital have a major voice in formulating policies that affect public relations, but they must assume their share of the task of informing the public regarding these policies. This cannot be left entirely to the administrator.

In addition to contacts with the public as patients, the emergency department has other opportunities to build good will. Three groups who frequent the department and carry away impressions are ambulance attendants, police, and representatives of the press.

AMBULANCE CREWS

It should be borne in mind that many ambulance attendants often have other duties that represent their major responsibilities.

Volunteer crews, which make up much of the ambulance service in New Jersey and some other states, take time from work or other activities with no reward other than the satisfaction of community service. All too often, the community fails to show appreciation. Fire department ambulance crews or those from other community services also need to get back to their main tasks. Promptness in admitting patients is important from the standpoint of freeing those ambulance attendants as well as from the standpoint of patient care. Young[2] states, "Nothing is more helpful to an ambulance crew than the prompt acceptance of its patient at the hospital nearest the scene of the emergency. Such acceptance results in the quickest possible medical care of the patient." Speaking of the delays or refusals in accepting accident victims, he continues, "Aside from the effects such delays may have on the patient, the ambulance and its crew are rendered ineffectual for the duration of the waiting period, and the crew remains responsible for the patient, who should be receiving medical attention."

Some interesting light was shed on this subject in the report of a project conducted by the North Carolina Hospital Education and Research Foundation, Inc., in cooperation with the Institute of Government and the Department of Hospital Administration of the School of Medicine of the University of North Carolina. This report, edited by Cadmus and Ketner,[3] says that 21 percent of the ambulance crews questioned stated that there was a delay in disposition of the patient "most of the time," and 54 percent stated there was a delay "some of the time." The crews were particularly critical of delays encountered at the hospitals associated with schools of medicine and at hospitals operated by an agency of the state or federal government. This interesting observation puts the community hospital in a better light than that in which some of its critics see it.

A transfer or exchange of property is often involved when a patient is brought by ambulance, and this should be expedited. Splints used on the patient should not be removed but should be exchanged for similar splints from the emergency department stockpile. The same procedure may involve sheets and blankets. Prearrangement of an understanding between the hospital and organizations operating ambulances in the community will avoid misunderstandings and speed up the exchange. Having these agreements in writing with copies on file in the emergency department will aid when new ambulance crews or new emergency department personnel are on duty.

POLICE

Not only do police often bring in the victims of accidents or other emergencies but they are responsible for obtaining all available information in connection with situations where legal liability may be involved. They are for the most part well disciplined and know where their responsibilities begin and end. They are deserving of the same cooperation and courtesy that they usually exhibit. They seldom interfere with patient care and are willing to wait until emergency measures have been taken before interviewing patients. When such measures have been taken, it is only reasonable that law enforcement officers be given the opportunity to gather information, as long as this is not injurious to the patient or does not delay further care. They will seldom take long to obtain the necessary data for their reports. As tentative diagnoses are called for in these reports, they should receive them. They are more concerned with the seriousness of injuries than with detailed anatomical diagnoses. Where fatalities have occurred, or may threaten, the actions of the police are influenced in such matters as holding those suspected of responsibility.

Policemen often prove helpful in handling unmanageable patients when the department is understaffed. Not only should they be treated with the respect due their positions, but their physical comforts should be provided for. A cup of hot coffee on a cold winter night will not hurt the public relations of the hospital. The same thoughts that were mentioned about conserving the time of ambulance crews apply to policemen. After all, their primary function is preservation of law and order, and they should not be delayed in this pursuit.

THE PRESS

While members of the press fall in an entirely different category from the police, they still deserve certain courtesies. It would be easy to claim that representatives of the press have no rights in the emergency department, for they certainly have no authority. They do have a responsibility to the public, and this involves getting the news. How they go about this will determine in each individual situation how much cooperation they may expect. Wherever possible, information should go out through the office of the administrator or his designated representative. Large hospitals having public relations departments will handle this problem in that way, but the majority of hospitals are not so highly organized. It should be recognized that the story will come out, so it might as well be accurate.

Bearing in mind the time-honored patient-physician relationship which involves privileged communications, there is still no point to a physician being secretive about the injuries to someone who was seen by a number of people at the roadside or elsewhere before he came to the hospital. On the other hand, the reporter who oversteps the bounds of good taste and seeks to outwit the emergency department attendants to get details that are neither his concern nor that of the public deserves to be rebuffed. A reporter was recently heard boasting of his "bag of tricks" used in evading the authorities in emergency departments. This same reporter, during the question period following a panel discussion on hospital emergencies, complained that the modern type of hospital emergency room construction, with several patients in one large room, made it difficult for him to "get a story" from a patient. He did not seem to realize that supplying news is not the primary function of such departments. Wise editors remove such reporters from hospital coverage and assign them to the waterfront or the police courts.

Experienced and cooperative reporters are usually satisfied with certain basic information which will include name, age, and address of the patient, his condition, and, if known, the name of the nearest relative. With this and the information he obtains outside the hospital, he can write a story that will be as complete as the average reader wishes. The name of the treating doctor may be requested, but he may not wish his name used, and most mature reporters will respect this wish.

Questions about the sobriety of the victim or the guilty one are not in the public interest at the moment. They should not be asked and if asked, should not be answered. Information obtained in the emergency department, whether given directly or through the administration, should emanate from the physicians and should not represent the opinions of nurses or others. A reporter trying to pry into too much detail should be told courteously but firmly that no more information will be available at the present. If he ever expects to get a story again, this should dampen his enthusiasm for details. If death has ensued, the coroner or the police are good sources to which to refer the press.

The press photographer falls in still another category. It is more difficult to defend his right even to be present than that of the man with the note pad and pencil. The photographer would be well advised to make his scoop where the cars are piled up. Still, there are times when a picture is part of the story. It is good practice to have the patient sign a consent form if he is amenable to being photographed. If he refuses, the photographer should be prohibited from taking the pictures. Otherwise there might be legal action against the hospital or doctor, although the photographer and his paper would really be the guilty ones.

If photographers come to the hospital and invade the privacy of patients, family, and friends in spite of admonitions against this, little time should be wasted in evicting them. If they represent responsible newspapers, they will seldom cause trouble. The free-lance photographer, who is responsible to no one, is more likely to be difficult to deal with. He may have a "bag of tricks."

It must be remembered that the news media may be a great asset to the hospital and its image. The hospital is in the business of trying to make sick people well. The newspaper or broadcasting station is in the business of gathering and disseminating the news. Both pursuits are praiseworthy. It will be in the public interest for those responsible for each to agree on certain ground rules before any misunderstandings arise. If this is done, misunderstandings may usually be avoided. Conferences between hospital administrators and newspaper editors can be most productive. These should be top-level affairs, at least they should start at the top level. If an editor later wants to designate one of his staff to such conferences, all well and good, but first the administrator should have the opportunity to make clear the position of the hospital to the highest authority on the newspaper. Then an agreement that will be beneficial to both institutions may be worked out. The result will be authoritative and dignified news from the hospital and well-planned and executed publicity for the hospital when it needs this.

Steps have been taken in a number of communities to establish working agreements between news media and hospitals. One example is the little brochure entitled *A guide to Ethical Hospital Press-TV-Radio Relationships* drawn up by the Chicago Hospital Council. Another similar and more recent agreement has been reached between the Michigan Hospital Association and the Michigan Press Association. These two documents present in a reasonable fashion the attitudes of both parties concerning the furnishing and obtaining of news about hospital patients.

THE CLERGY

Regardless of the beliefs of the physician in charge, he is narrowminded to the point of stupidity if he does not recognize the value of a clergyman of the patient's faith when the patient is in a critical condition. Every effort should be made to provide an opportunity for minister, priest, or rabbi to offer spiritual comfort to the severely injured or otherwise critically ill patient. This is not a matter of public relations but of human relations, the value of which is appreciated by any well-rounded member of the medical profession.

LAWYERS

Lawyers have the same rights, of course, as other friends and relatives of the patients, but not in their professional capacity. With patients or their relatives under the stress of recent happenings, this is no time to take statements relating to settlements. The facts will not change, and the time for legal discussions is when the situations have been assessed and reasonable prognoses may be made. The ethics of the legal profession does not allow this immediate postaccident activity, and it will seldom be necessary to take steps to prevent it in most communities.

Members of the legal profession should have a close relationship to the entire emergency department program but not on the spot at the time of the emergency. There are many features of the program calling for policy decisions that should have legal backing. Such matters are as follows:

The responsibility of the hospital to provide *actual treatment* for nonemergency conditions in the emergency department.

Responsibility to arrange for follow-up care.

The matter of implied consent vs signed permission for treatment.

Consent for minors when parents or other responsible adults are not present.

Control of privileges, based on training and experience, of individual members of the medical staff working in the emergency department.

Refusal of patients to agree to treatment advised by medical staff members.

Responsibility for notifying health authorities or police in accordance with the law.

These are only some of the areas in which disagreement and litigation might arise. Such situations should be included in the manual of policies and procedures with specific directions as to the action to be taken. The courts are usually sensitive to whether the stated procedures have been carried out in any department of a hospital.

Public relations in the emergency department are based on the same principles as such relations elsewhere in the institution. Hospitals are complex organizations and becoming more so. They must, perforce, set policies and establish rules, the reasons for which are not always self-evident. Many a newly elected hospital trustee requires a considerable period of indoctrination before he appreciates some of the procedures. When he finally does, he should be the first to recognize that those on the outside may naturally and quite honestly question hospital policies. When the public buys hospital services today, it does not see many low price tags. It is paying a good price and deserves to know what it is buying. A wise governing board will make sure that the public is informed regarding carefully established policies and changes in policies. This is the real foundation of public relations. It should not be forgotten that there may be a difference between "good" public relations and "sound" public relations. The latter will stand the test of time.

REFERENCES

1. Rusk, H.A.: Barrier for medicare. *New York Times*, Aug. 8, 1965.
2. Young, C.B., Jr.: *Transportation of the Injured*. Springfield, Thomas, pp. 215–216.
3. Cadmus, R.R., and Ketner, J.H.: Organizing Ambulance Services in the Public Interest, 1965.

Chapter 14

PEOPLE AND PROBLEMS

The emergency department of a general hospital is neither easy to administer nor to work in. Many factors contribute to this, but they are mostly concerned with people. This chapter will concern itself with some of these people. It should be obvious that these problems perpetrated by people will follow no pattern.

Although the administrator, the directress of nurses, and the physician members of an emergency department committee have agreed on general principles and want to conduct the most efficient program possible, they should realize that problems will constantly arise and thought must be given to their solution. Some of the people who will not add to the smoothness of the operation are the following:

1. The *physician* who objects to taking his turn on a rotating roster. If his reason is frankly one of inadequacy, he is probably right. Leaving him off may be in the best interests of the patients. If it is unwillingness to make the effort or give the time, it can be labeled selfishness. The burden of proof should be on him to support his refusal. This problem has been mentioned in the chapter on staffing. There is a limit to how much a hospital owes a doctor without some return support.

2. The *physician* who is chronically late in answering calls. Reasonable delays may be overlooked unless the doctor has been informed that the situation is so serious as to demand his immediate attendance. Repeated tardiness is ample reason for inquiry by the chairman of the emergency department committee or a department chief if the director is not able to solve the problem.

In this connection, it is well to state here that it is not wise to include in a procedure manual a rule stating a specific time limit within which doctors should respond to calls. When the

Executive Committee of the Committee on Trauma of the American College of Surgeons was revising its standards in 1964, the author, who was at that time Secretary for the Committee, urged that the 15-minute arrival clause be removed, but he was overruled. Later that year, the Joint Commission on Accreditation of Hospitals accepted the Trauma Committee's wording when it published its *Standards for Emergency Departments.* The Commission[1] has since then seen the danger in this and changed the wording to read "within a reasonable time" instead of a specific time. It explains this and other changes by saying, "In addition some specific language often fails to win the approval of legal advisors, on the principle that specificity increases liability." The College of Surgeons has now adopted the Commission's revised *Standards,* so it no longer includes the 15-minute clause. It is astounding how some people need a lawyer to point out something that is self-evident. The inclusion of the 15-minute requirement was an invitation to a lawyer for the plaintiff to claim neglect if the record showed that the doctor did not arrive until 20 minutes after he was called in a case where the end result was less than hoped for.

3. The *physician* who fails to be available when he is on call. In communities where general practitioners man the emergency department at least part of the time, they will devote some of their practice to house calls. When doing this, they should keep their offices or the hospital informed of their itinerary so they may be reached promptly. The doctor on second call has the same responsibility, within reasonable limits. If the man on first call knows that he will be unavailable for certain periods of time, it should be his responsibility to make sure that the man on second call is available. It is particularly important that a surgeon on the roster be available.

4. The *physician* who neglects the completion of records. This type of doctor is one that every hospital staff must contend with. While his failure to keep his records up to date on inpatients may be a matter of administrative deficiency, his failure in the emergency department should not be tolerated. He loses the opportunity to keep an accurate record if he doesn't write it up at the time. Many of these patients he will not see again, and the

record has legal as well as professional implications. This has been elaborated upon in the chapters on medical records and on legal aspects.

5. The *nurse* who fails to rise to the occasion when confronted with above-average responsibilities can be a problem. In Chapter 7 on staffing, the characteristics of the ideal emergency department nurse are mentioned. She will, on occasion, have to make decisions not called for in other places and do things that nurses don't usually have to do. A nurse who cannot adapt to this environment will sooner or later become a liability and should be assigned to tasks more in line with her talents and desires.

6. The *adult patient* who, for reasons only he would accept, refuses proper treatment. There are many such situations. These may occur in partially intoxicated patients who are temporarily devoid of judgment. It may be a matter of a patient minimizing his injuries. He may refuse to have a laceration sutured with some such statement as, "Oh, Doc, just tape it up." He may refuse an x-ray of a possibly fractured ankle, demanding only an elastic bandage so that he may walk out. He may refuse tetanus immunization because he "doesn't like needles." The latter refusal is more likely to come from a parent in the case of a child. Fortunately, the parents who "do not believe in shots" are becoming fewer and fewer.

In any of these situations involving refusal of treatment, the physician should request the patient or the parent to sign a release of responsibility for both doctor and hospital. Forms should be available for this. In the rare cases where both treatment and signature are refused (and this does happen), the facts should be clearly recorded on the record and signed by both doctor and nurse. Patients have been known to change their minds when they see this being done.

7. The *child* who refuses necessary treatment. This will present a problem that will tax the patience of any doctor. The presence of a sensible parent will usually suffice to bring the little patient to terms, albeit without enthusiasm. Occasionally, a parent will side with the child. If an appeal to reason does not cause him or her to capitulate, the release form is next in order.

Where a proposed treatment, such as suturing a laceration, would be painful, the parent may in all seriousness ask, "Won't you put something on it so it won't hurt?" She (it is usually the mother) may already have made a verbal contract with the child that the doctor won't hurt him (it is usually a boy!). How to break that contract without the mother losing face may not be easy. An explanation to the mother that the only way to completely prevent pain would be to put the child to sleep frequently succeeds, particularly if it is accompanied by a description of severe nausea and vomiting during the recovery period. If the mother has never been the recipient of one of our current pleasant anesthetics, completely devoid of all discomfort and distress, she will probably decide that it is time to take a firm stand and let the doctor get on with his business.

8. *Members of family* of sick or injured. No hard and fast rule will apply to every situation. Unless the treatment area is crowded with patients, a limited number of relatives may be allowed in for very short periods and these only in an effort to reassure patients, particularly minors, and to provide useful information. Relatives may insist on staying, but this should not be allowed except in the most unusual circumstances. Even children will usually cooperate after a parent has seen them settled on a treatment stretcher and reassured them that he or she will be waiting nearby. In those rare cases, such as mentioned in the previous paragraph, no progress will be made in the absence of a parent or other relative.

9. *Friends* of the injured or others involved in the accident. These people may be a real problem. Sometimes through a feeling of guilt they will assume practically a possessive attitude toward the patient and give the impression that they must supervise the care. Difficult as it may be, some patience should be shown with them, remembering that they may be distraught to the point of irresponsibility. In the end, they may have to be evicted from the room. If they leave voluntarily, the situation will be better. In large departments where personnel is not limited, there is usually someone who is able to deal with these unwanted observers. In smaller hospitals where possibly one doctor and one nurse are handling the whole situation, they will

not have time to devote to policing the area. This is one reason why hard and fast rules are not practical. Frequently one or more bystanders will be calm enough to understand the problem and aid in calming others and taking them to the waiting room. Of course, under no circumstances should anyone be allowed in the operating room, other than patient and hospital personnel.

10. *Reporters* and *photographers* may get out of line, although the more experienced and responsible ones are less likely to. Restrictions on them are discussed in the chapter on public relations.

11. A rare troublemaker, but one occasionally seen, particularly in large cities, is the out-and-out *gangster* or *criminal*. He may be the patient, or he may accompany the patient. These men sometimes take complete command. They may issue threats. They may refuse to give any history or any other information that will aid in the diagnosis. This may be to cover their own guilt or to protect them from retaliation. They may in certain instances dictate the treatment, as some of them are not without previous experience in accident situations. In the absence of police protection and where it is obvious that characters of this type are being dealt with, it is advisable to do as little talking as possible, provide the necessary treatment, and allow them to go their way. Nothing will be gained and much may be lost by exhibiting an antagonistic or threatening attitude toward them. Of course, if an attendant recognizes the situation and can get to a telephone out of hearing, the police may be called. I have been threatened in an emergency department, but never injured, and to my knowledge, have never aided a fugitive from justice.

12. *Prisoners* already in the custody of the law may be brought to the hospital for emergency treatment. In such cases, it is advisable to allow the law enforcement officer to stand by during treatment.

The larger and more completely staffed emergency departments will be better able to deal with uncooperative people, but problems may arise anywhere. It must be borne in mind that emotions may be at high pitch, and more than an average amount of tact and understanding may be required. It goes without saying that the highest priority belongs to the proper care of the sick or injured, and when troublesome bystanders threaten to interfere with this, firmness is required.

13. Members of the *lay public* may for a variety of reasons present problems. Whether they have been patients or not, they may choose to criticize the department, sometimes fairly but more often unfairly. Their criticisms must be dealt with reasonably but not defensively. This whole book is designed to recommend methods of operating the department in a way to decrease the vulnerability to fair criticism. In the previous chapter on public relations, there are discussions bearing on this.

14. Occasionally, members of the *Board of Trustees* may receive complaints about the emergency department or other departments of the hospital. Their friends, knowing of their connections with the hospital, may come to them with their grievances. By the time these complaints, often starting at social events, reach those responsible for the departments, the facts may be so diluted with fiction that it may be very difficult to identify the incidents concerned. If a member of the Board of Trustees has served on the planning committee that established the departmental policies, he can assist in mollifying his fellow member. Although he need not remain on the committee that is responsible for the functioning of the department, he can probably be counted on for helpful support. Hospital trustees are legally as well as morally responsible for the quality of care in all departments of the hospital. For this reason, it is to be expected that they will want to know the facts about incidents that result in complaints. It is to be hoped, however, that they will not prejudge those responsible for emergency department care, or for that matter care in any department, and that if they do find the criticism is unfair will be as eager to seek out the complainant as he was to come to them. The hospital trustee should consider himself a member of the health care team and, as such, should support his teammates unless they are obviously making errors.

REFERENCE

1. Joint Commission on Accreditation of Hospitals. Bulletin 48, April 1968.

Chapter 15

FOR DOCTORS ONLY—
PARTICULARLY SURGEONS

It is interesting to note the changing attitudes of the public and the members of the profession toward various pursuits in the healing art. Whereas the surgeon today seems to be surrounded by an aura that makes him the object of envy, this was not always true. One need only look back about two centuries in medical history to find the surgeon as a man with much inferior education and thus a lower social status than his medical confrère. As a matter of fact, the two were scarcely confrères. In the British Isles, an aspirant to the practice of medicine took a classical education at a university and usually followed this with the study of medicine on the Continent. The youth aspiring to become a surgeon attached himself to someone practicing surgery, without first obtaining a cultural education. If he applied himself and proved to have some ability, the Barber-Surgeons Company recognized him at the end of seven years and granted him the privilege of practicing under certain restrictions laid down by the company.

To digress for a moment, it is interesting to note that although these young men were usually not cultured, there were at least some requirements for their acceptance into the surgical guild, requirements based on training apart from that demanded of physicians. To this day, our licensing authorities in the United States have not seen fit to require any training over and above that obtained by the general physician, for the granting of a license to practice medicine and *surgery*. Much of the friction between doctors and the surgical departments of hospitals, as well as the reported performance of surgical operations by the untrained, could be wiped out overnight by bringing our licensing practices up to date.

The surgeons of Great Britain have long since escaped their low status in life and have set themselves apart from the rest of the medical profession by disdaining to use the title of "Doctor." They become doctors of medicine and then when they have completed their postdoctoral training as surgeons, call themselves "Mister." This I have heard referred to by a former president of one of the Royal Colleges of Surgeons as "snobbery in reverse."

The recognition of adequate surgical training in this country by the various certifying boards and colleges has had a good effect on the quality of American surgery. More and more hospitals are beginning to require an acceptable amount of formal surgical training before granting operating privileges to new applicants. Even patients are, in some instances, making inquiry about the training of a surgeon before submitting to his administrations. There is little doubt that this movement toward limiting the practice of surgery to trained surgeons could go ahead at a more rapid pace if all those in a position to influence it would speak out. Their lack of support is difficult to understand, but the movement is in the right direction, and it is to be hoped that it will continue.

There are usually some bad effects in the train of any forward movement, and this trend toward superior training in American surgery is no exception. The aura referred to above that surrounds the well-trained surgeon of today is partially the result of his having become a performer of miracles. All too often during his training, the young surgeon jumps from the field of basic surgical sciences into an arena where the spotlight is focused on exotic and often rare surgical procedures. He misses that phase in his training experience that surgeons of past generations went through, the care of injuries. He all too often regards this area of surgery as beneath him. Such things seldom add luster to his image, and he fails to see in them a great opportunity to serve many of his fellow men in need. Doctors and particularly surgeons are often accused of centering their professional planning on material gain. Granting that there is some truth in this, it is the opinion of the author that more often surgeons strive for prestige. That the latter can later lead to increased income cannot be denied, but many members of the profession think more of their status than they do of their bank accounts, even in later years.

The cleaning and repair of wounds, the setting of fractures, the management of shock, the treating of acute poisoning, and other things required in the day-in and day-out practice of medicine and surgery in the emergency department of a hospital offer a challenge that is difficult to equal. Among other things, they offer the opportunity for excellence. To consider such things as secondary in importance to the type of complaints requiring repeated home or office visits, or in-hospital treatment, is to exhibit a warped view of human need. If a physician is not willing to give his best or to prepare himself to render superior care in the emergency department, it is reasonable to doubt if he is deserving of full confidence elsewhere. The prevention of prolonged infection and disfiguring scars by the skilled and meticulous care of an open wound can be a source of satisfaction and pride. The proper reduction of a fracture resulting in full function of an extremity, rather than a "good enough" result will bring gratitude from almost any patient. Here in the emergency department, the physician who may not possess all of the certificates that some of his colleagues may have has the opportunity to show his true worth. This should not be interpreted as a suggestion that staff members of limited training attempt things beyond their abilities. Willingness to admit the need of help is one of the hallmarks of a trustworthy physician. Men who have that hallmark will need little supervision unless they call for it.

As noted in Chapter 7, full-time emergency department practice bids fair to become a recognized specialty. When it does, let us hope that it will appeal to some of our most capable young physicians. Many argue that all surgery should be done only by fully trained surgeons. There are sound reasons to support this stand, but in actual practice it does not work out in many emergency departments. Surgical schedules and the attitude of some surgeons demand that others must carry out some of the procedures in the emergency department. A good training in general medicine and in the surgery of trauma will fit a doctor for capable work in this field. Those willing to take such training and who show an interest in this type of work should be encouraged. They will find it rewarding, not only in satisfaction but in a material way as well. Some who have entered this field on a full-time basis, with some misgivings, have been pleasantly surprised at their incomes.

The tendency to downgrade practice in this area has been emphasized by Mason,[1] who says, "A study of emergency rooms made elsewhere has shown that in general they are not too well staffed and organized for the job they have to do. Equipment and supplies are lacking, personnel are not properly instructed and too often the emergency department is looked upon as a sort of gratuitous training ground where the inexperienced junior intern learns to put in stitches or to pump out the stomach of a suspected victim of poisoning. Although situations in the emergency room often demand the most experienced and careful judgment possible, they are often left to the hands of the youngest and least experienced. Too often the explanation for leaving an emergency to the junior intern as a training for him has been an excuse for avoiding a disagreeable task which came at an inconvenient time."

It is emphasized in Chapter 18 that the emergency department is a good place for the intern to learn, but not by the trial-and-error method. The idea that interns can take care of patients coming to the emergency department because they are not very important people is of course at variance with the basic concepts of good medical practice. As has been noted elsewhere,[2] we should not strive for a better end result in one patient than in another because one person is more important than the other. The lack of appreciation shown by some patients for a valiant effort to restore them to normal and their lack of cooperation is often discouraging to say the least, but no excuse for lessening the effort. We must agree with Theseus[3] in *A Midsummer-Night's Dream*, who remarks, "With the help of a surgeon, he might yet recover and prove an ass," but we cannot be sure of this. He might turn out to be a valuable member of society, and it is our duty to give him every assistance toward that end. Perhaps Rhoads, Allen, Harkins, and Moyer[4] included the emergency department in their thinking when they said with relation to hospital duties, "The unpopular assignments are often the ones where good performance will stand out most and be most appreciated."

The primary purpose of this book is to discuss the planning, building, equipping, and operation of a department of a hospital. However, since the purpose of the entire effort is patient care, it does not seem inappropriate to include a brief discussion of some points concerned with this, particularly from the standpoint of accidental injuries.

Some of the things to which the capable emergency department physician should direct his attention are mentioned in the following.

COMPLETE EXAMINATION OF THE PATIENT

It cannot be stressed too often that the most serious aspects of accidental injuries may not, particularly at first, produce the most noticeable signs or symptoms. Any trauma that damages one part of the body may damage others. The "multiple injury patient" may not know that he has multiple injuries. He deserves a complete survey by the first physician to attend him. Preoccupation with one injury may lead to neglect of a more serious injury. Wilson, Vidrine, and Rives[5] have emphasized this in the case of abdominal injuries accompanied by head injuries. They mention not only the preoccupation with the head injury, but the fact that symptoms of the abdominal injury may be misinterpreted and wrongly ascribed to cerebral damage. They report a mortality rate for blunt abdominal trauma four times greater when it is accompanied by head injury. Even though a patient may be in coma from a head injury, abdominal rigidity or lack of peristaltic sounds should not be attributed to this. Intra-abdominal injury must be considered.

Granted that such emergencies as compression pneumothorax, active bleeding, or any other obvious emergency should have first attention, no time should be lost after this in making a complete examination of the patient.

SHOCK

One of the most serious conditions to be dealt with in any emergency department is shock. It is one of the prime causes of death following severe injury. The necessity for recognizing this condition, particularly its early manifestations, is one of the reasons why the selection and training of personnel is so important. Thinking beyond the actual signs and symptoms is required. The history of the injury often gives a clue to what may be expected. Physicians treating air-raid casualties in Britain in World War II learned to anticipate shock from certain injuries or combinations of injuries before the actual signs appeared. Vaughan[6] stated in this connection, "The only real guide to treatment is seriousness of the injury, regardless of hemoconcentration. Regardless of a normal blood pressure don't send the seriously injured to the operating room, without a transfusion or they will have a serious collapse."

These things do not require specialty training. This is just good practical general medicine—dramatic, but not highly technical. Further discussion of shock will be found in Chapter 11 on Hospital Disaster Plans. A point that is sometimes forgotten in the management of patients suffering from shock following hemorrhage or from other causes is the careful recording of the patient's progress or lack of it. This is important in preparing him for surgery and in deciding if he is a fit candidate for surgery. The memory should not be trusted. Records of vital signs should be recorded at periodic intervals so there will be no guesswork about the course of the patient's condition. Clinical impressions should be recorded along with blood pressure, pulse, respirations, and laboratory determinations. These repeated clinical notations during the critical minutes or hours are best made by the same person. It may be difficult for one physician to communicate his impression to another. This indicates the need for doctors remaining with seriously injured patients, particularly those with impending shock.

In disaster planning, where it may be anticipated that there will be many shock patients, it cannot be too strongly emphasized that surgeons of experience are needed in the triage area. Prompt and definite decisions must be made there and priorities determined.

CARDIAC ARREST

There is no emergency calling for more prompt and positive action than cessation of heart beat. It must be understood that even the most skilled prompt attention will not reactivate every heart that has stopped beating. Some of the publicity that has been given regarding cardiac compression has not been in the public interest. It has led some people to expect too much. Where it is evident that massive injury has resulted in death, it may be self-evident that any attempt at cardiac resuscitation would be doomed to failure. However, if there is any hope of success, it should be attempted. External cardiac compression is a technique that should be taught to all professional personnel in emergency departments. Excellent posters with clearly described illustrations of the technique are available and should be on the wall. If cardiac action is not restored within four minutes, the patient will probably never be normal even though he survives. It must be remembered that artificial respiration is needed along with restoration of heart beat.

ASPHYXIA

While not as difficult to treat or as alarming as cardiac arrest, failure to breathe will be just as fatal if not treated promptly. Even though artificial respiration by first-aid methods without mechanical equipment may be called for outside the hospital, every emergency department should have resuscitation equipment available at all times. Here again, the technique is not difficult, but the time to read the directions is not just before the equipment is used. All doctors and nurses who may be called upon to treat emergency department patients should know how to use the available equipment correctly and promptly. Such equipment is described in Chapter 5.

FRACTURES

Good care of fractures in an emergency department or any-where else depends mainly on two things—a knowledge of certain fundamentals and a good conscience. The former should make it possible for many doctors of medicine to reduce fractures well and hold them in position. The latter will cause them to ask for more experienced help if their efforts have not been successful. The important thing is not the classification of the doctor or what board certificate he has, but whether he is willing and has the patience to apply the fundamentals. He should either take an interest in fractures and treat them well or always refer the patient to someone else.

There is no question that surgeons, if they are completely trained, will provide better fracture care than most general practitioners, but this does not mean that some general practitioners cannot do excellent work in this field. This applies particularly to such things as Colle's fractures, fractures of the shaft of the humerus, and even the tibia and fibula. Fewer of them will be able to handle fractures of the femur, forearm, or even fingers, which may be among the most difficult to reduce and hold in place.

Arguments as to whether orthopedists or general surgeons should care for fractures in a hospital are silly. It is the training and interest, not the title, that counts. Many capable and conservative general surgeons will provide better fracture care than radical orthopedists. Criticisms of general surgeons being "too quick with the knife" are heard and sometimes well justified. By the same token, some orthopedists are "too quick with the screwdriver." There is no more reason to rule general surgeons out of the care of broken bones than there is to prevent the orthopedist from treating wounds. The last restriction would take from him open fractures. However, no one can deny that in all too many general surgical training programs, fracture care is almost completely neglected. These trainees are not fit to care for fractures; in fact, they cannot do it as well as some general practitioners. The reason for this may be a lack of interest or knowledge on the part of their trainers. It may also be due to a hospital regulation that all the fractures go to the orthopedic service. The latter is evidence of the current tendency toward overspecialization.

FRACTURE FUNDAMENTALS

The first consideration in the care of fractures in the emergency department is the prevention of further damage. Splinting at the scene of the accident is improving but not as rapidly as it should. All emergency department personnel should be versed in this and should apply splints immediately, particularly to lower extremity fractures, if this has not been done previously. The splints should stay in place during the time the x-rays are being taken and until the definite treatment is begun. In long-bone fractures, it should not be forgotten that traction is the fundamental maneuver. It prevents soft tissue damage, relieves pain, and often reduces the fracture. A discussion of the definitive care of the many types of fractures is not appropriate to a work of this type, but the above fundamentals plus extreme care in dealing with fractures of the neck and spine are the basis of competent fracture care. There is no better short treatise on the subject than the *Fracture Manual of the Committee on Trauma of the American College of Surgeons.* It should be present in every emergency department.

WOUND CARE

The attempt to destroy bacteria in an open wound by the introduction of antiseptics such as iodine or merthiolate is the stamp of antiquity on any physician. The idea that a wound is infected because it is soiled is unfortunately too often entertained. Such wounds are not infected until the bacteria begin to multiply and penetrate. The best guard against this is their early removal. This is a mechanical procedure, not difficult but requiring prompt and positive action. It is because of this that such things as open fractures should take precedence over such things as acute appendicitis among emergency operations. This may require a bit of convincing with some surgeons, but it is in line with the philosophy that emergency department patients are not second-class. In acute appendicitis the infection is already established, and with proper preoperative management a delay of an hour or two will make little difference. In the case of the open fracture, the delay may convert contamination to established infection.

After the surrounding skin is thoroughly cleaned, bacteria are removed from a wound by excision of damaged and soiled tissue and copious irrigation with saline solution. The amount of tissue to be removed will be determined by the judgment of the operator. Torn or crushed muscle whose vascularity has been lost will not regenerate and will only act as a culture medium if left. As the wound is irrigated, this damaged tissue will have a pale appearance in contrast to healthy viable muscle. Torn or shredded fascia is also of no value. Such tissue should be excised either with a scalpel or very sharp scissors. When tissue is being excised, any foreign bodies such as cinders, gravel, clothing, or splinters should be removed. This also applies to small fragments of bone that have become completely detached from their periosteum. Larger fragments of bone, the absence of which would compromise the establishment of firm bony union, should best be preserved but should be thoroughly cleaned. Irrigation by sterile saline is done intermittently during the removal of devitalized tissue and foreign bodies. In deep wounds, this should be done from the depth of the wound out. A glass tip delivering saline by gravity through tubing from a flask should be inserted deep in the wound so that foreign material will be washed out of and not into the wound. The irrigation of wounds involving fractures is similar to that involving only soft tissues but requires more care to be sure that all contaminated areas lateral to and beneath the bone are reached.

Except on the face and on extensor surfaces over joints, where loss of skin cannot be afforded, the excision of a narrow strip of skin from the margins of the wound will usually be advisable. The cut edges of the skin may be contaminated or crushed and in either case may not heal by primary union when the wound is sutured. On the face or forehead, the blood supply is so adequate that if the skin is viable it will usually heal without excising the edges.

After any wound is cleaned, a decision must be made with regard to primary closure. The deciding factors will be the amount of contamination, the time that has elapsed since wounding, and the desirability of striving for primary union with a minimum of scarring. These are matters of experience and difficult to describe. If the successful cleaning of the wound is doubtful, it may best be left open. Secondary closure after a few days is not difficult and if infection has not developed, little time will be lost in ultimate healing. Although the toilet of wounds complicating fractures has been described here, these will seldom be treated in the emergency department. The care of "compound" fractures is major surgery.

Thorough hemostasis is also a prerequisite to primary union. Hematomas not only prevent apposition of approximated tissues but provide culture media. Ligation of bleeding vessels and compression without constriction are the best guards against post-repair bleeding. "Kling" bandage will provide pressure on the dressing without constriction.

The splinting of some wounds is indicated even though not accompanied by fracture. This applies particularly to wounds over joints, where motion of the joint might interfere with primary healing.

Prophylaxis against infection in wounds may also be augmented by the judicious use of appropriate antibiotics, but they are no substitute for thorough wound cleaning. If the bacteria are removed, little antibiotic or chemotherapy will be needed. Prophylaxis against tetanus should be a matter of staff decision, and the proper procedures should be outlined in the department policy manual. An excellent poster on this subject has been prepared by the Committee on Trauma of the American College of Surgeons and is available for posting in emergency departments by writing to the American College of Surgeons.

BURNS

Burns of slight intensity or of limited areas are seldom dangerous. Extensive burns of second or third degree require prompt admission to the hospital and systemic as well as local treatment.

Further discussion of burns will be found in Chapter 11. A poster outling well-accepted methods in the emergency treatment of burns has also been published by the American College of Surgeons. It was prepared by the Subcommittee on Burns of the Committee on Trauma and is also available from the American College of Surgeons.

The foregoing features of emergency department practice have not been presented with any idea that they are completely covered from a clinical standpoint. They have been outlined to call attention to the fact that emergency department treatment is not of secondary importance and is worthy of the best efforts of any doctor of medicine. The prevention of death and permanent disability offers challenges equal to those in any field of medicine. The emergency department is where these challenges are constantly faced.

REFERENCES

1. Mason, M.L.: *Am J Surgery,* 97:4, p. 411, 1959.
2. Spencer, J.H.: Please call a doctor. *Bull Am Coll Surgeons,* 39:119–124, 1954.
3. Shakespeare, Wm.: *A Midsummer-Night's Dream,* Act V, Scene I.
4. Rhoads, J.E., Allen, J.G., Harkins, H.N., and Moyer, C.A.: *Surgery—Principles and Practice.* Philadelphia, Lippincott, p. 5, 1957.
5. Wilson, C.B., Vidrine, A., Jr., and Rives, J.D.: Coexistent head and abdominal injury. *Ann Surg, 161:*608–613, 1965.
6. Vaughan, Janet, M.D., F.R.C.P.: Personal communication in course in war surgery taken by the writer at Hammersmith Hospital, London, 1943.

Chapter 16

MEDICAL EMERGENCIES

I. THE CARDIAC RECEIVING ROOM
AND PREHOSPITAL CARDIAC CARE*

RICHARD S. CRAMPTON

INTRODUCTION

Organizing, equipping, staffing, and supervising the cardiac receiving room of the emergency department will necessarily reflect the size of the hospital, community, and professional staff. No matter what the limitations imposed by the size of the hospital and community, by the ambulance system, and by the number of doctors and nurses available, emergency service should always incorporate early identification and treatment of the patient with a cardiac crisis.[1] The highest priority is the diagnosis and treatment of dysrhythmias in order to prevent the need for resuscitation.[2] Dysrhythmias in the clinical settings of acute myocardial ischemia, sinus arrest or heart block due to fibrosclerosis of the conduction system, and digitalis sensitivity may cause sudden catastrophe and are particularly rewarding when prevented or treated promptly.[3] All the equipment and medications of a comprehensive cardiac care unit should be kept in the cardiac receiving room. An emergency telephone information center should be created connecting the emergency department, the coronary care or intensive care unit, the rescue squad or ambulance service, and in small communities the physician's home and office.[4] Thus, patients

* The author thanks the Charles A. Frueaff Foundation, Inc., of New York City and the teen-age cast of the Christian folk musical, *Natural High*, for financing equipment of the Mobile Coronary Care Unit, Department of Medicine, University of Virginia Medical Center; and Heart Attack Rescue Service, Charlottesville-Albemarle Rescue Squad.

243

suddenly in distress from cardiac emergencies may call for help and receive prompt treatment from a cardiac ambulance team designed to function as an arm of the emergency department of the hospital which can be tailored to suit the needs of any type of community.[1,5,6,7]

ELECTRICAL SAFETY AND CHOOSING EQUIPMENT

Protection from electrical hazards by a carefully constructed cardiac receiving room, by soundly designed equipment, by careful use of equipment, and by regular inspection as part of a program of preventive maintenance is necessary for the safety of the patient and for the safety of those caring for the patient.[8] In hospitals where an electrical or biomedical engineer is available, these professionals should be included in all plans for buying new equipment or updating existing equipment. Consultation with a biomedical engineer outside the hospital should be sought if none is available in the hospital or community. The type of equipment must suit the needs of each particular hospital and community. Purchase of new equipment should not be left to chance or to the whims of unsophisticated hospital administrators, nurses, physicians, and surgeons. Consultation and discussion amongst the nursing and medical staffs and engineers aware of the practical and intellectual limitations of the clinical staff using and abusing electrical monitoring, recording, and lifesaving equipment is needed so that the safest, most practical equipment for the needs of the cardiac patient can be bought.

The cardiac receiving room should have a generous supply of three-pin grounding, electrical wall receptacles for 110-volt AC current. The ground pin of each receptacle should be directly attached to a third ground wire brought through the electrical conduit, and mechanical bonding of conduits, armored cables, and receptacles to their respective boxes must not be relied upon for ground. The conduit should contain the three wires: high, neutral, and ground. There should be a common ground for all electrical equipment in the cardiac receiving room if it serves a single patient, or for each patient monitoring area in a larger cardiac observation room. Since improperly wired AC wall receptacles present a variety of serious electrical hazards, each receptacle should be inspected regularly for reversed neutral and high polarity, improper ground, improper neutral, reversed ground and power, and a minimum release force or tension of 8 to 10 oz. Receptacles providing 220-volt AC current for portable x-ray equipment should be of the four-pin type and likewise need regular inspection. Like other critical care areas such as operating, delivery, and recovery rooms, and intensive and coronary care units, the receptacles providing power for the equipment of the emergency department and cardiac receiving room should be connected to the hospital's emergency power system for instant transfer in the event of a hospital or community power failure.

The choice of equipment should be tempered by a number of considerations: electrical safety, simplicity, reliability, ease of use, rapid repair, and easy maintenance. Since extreme electrical hazards to the patient and hospital personnel exist with two-wire power cords, instruments and equipment should not be bought or used until a three-wire power cord with grounding of the chassis of the apparatus has been connected. This common sense rule applies to all AC-powered electrical equipment, ranging from cardiac defibrillators to floor lamps. When buying new electrical instruments or equipment from the manufacturer or distributor, the hospital purchasing office must insist upon three-wire power cords with proper grounding. Each piece of new or updated equipment must be checked for safety upon receipt and before clinical use. Once the cardiac receiving room and its equipment have been assembled, an environmental electrical safety check must be carried out before use and at regular intervals thereafter. In particular, tests must be conducted for leakage of current from instruments, equipment, electrical appliances, and metal furniture due to broken or poorly connected grounds, due to leaks exceeding the high or low range of the manufacturer's specifications by way of the ground, or due to loss of "isolation" of the instrument from the patient. Electrical beds are a dangerous luxury and should not be used in the cardiac receiving room or any other critical care area.*

EQUIPMENT

In cardiac emergency work, the most versatile, safe, mobile equipment is battery-powered. These virtues of battery power allow instant use at the patient's side anywhere in the cardiac receiving room, emergency department, hospital, and outside the hospital. Such equipment can also be used during an episode of hospital power failure. One drawback of battery-powered equipment is keeping it charged, which requires meticulous attention and regular inspection from responsible people, particularly after each episode of use. Another disadvantage is the small size of the oscilloscopes. Some battery-powered equipment is designed to operate from an AC power source as an alternative. However, the safety from electrical hazards declines where equipment attached to the patient is connected to AC power. Furthermore, in prehospital cardiac care, one cannot rely upon finding an appropriate AC receptacle to provide power for emergency equipment. Although ambulances can be equipped to provide AC current, it may not be feasible due to clinical circumstances to move a critically ill patient to the ambulance and have the patient survive. For example, if ventricular fibrillation is encountered in the house, office, factory, football stadium, or other place where a heart attack may occur, the best treatment is prompt cardiac defibrillation on the spot, supplemented by cardiopulmonary resuscitation.[9] The former cannot be accomplished without a defibrillator, and the latter is very difficult to conduct effectively during transfer of the pulseless, apneic patient from the site of the cardiac arrest through halls, stairways, elevators, and ramps to the ambulance containing a cardiac defibrillator.

One of the best examples of versatile battery-powered

* Hospital administrators would be well advised to develop a critical attitude toward many labor-saving devices. The introduction of dangerous equipment to save muscle power is not good administration.—JHS

equipment is the cardiac monitor-defibrillator made by Physio Control, Seattle, Washington. The unit comes in a strong case and is the only one satisfying military specifications. Instant detection and monitoring of the cardiac rhythm is provided by electrocardiographic electrodes contained in the defibrillator paddles which are placed on the chest over the lower sternum and cardiac apex. The rhythm of the heart is observed on the oscilloscope (Fig. 37). If ventricular fibrillation is detected, it takes 15 seconds to charge up and deliver a 400-watt-second direct current shock. This defibrillator delivers up to 40 un-synchronized direct-current shocks at the 400-watt-second level of energy before complete discharge of its battery. How-

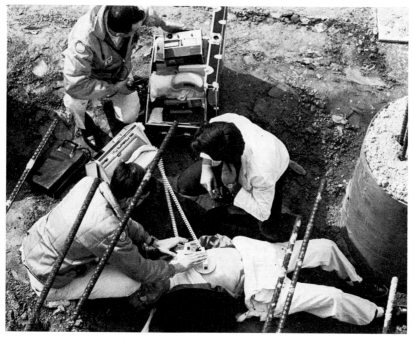

Figure 37. Prehospital coronary care. The rescue worker has placed the monitor-defibrillator paddles over the heart of a construction worker who collapsed at work from a heart attack. The physician is observing the cardiac rhythm on the oscilloscope. The second rescue worker is preparing the electrocardiograph and its electrodes to obtain a diagnostic twelve-lead record. An intravenous drip should be started. (Courtesy of the *Charlottesville Daily Progress*.)

ever, a quick-charging system capable of restoring the completely discharged battery in 15 minutes is available from Biocom, Culver City, California, if the purchaser requests that the Physio Control monitor-defibrillator be shipped from Seattle via Culver City to his hospital. Several other options are worth adding, including a built-in testing system for the adequacy of the level of electrical energy delivered; a swiveling, collapsible intravenous pole for portable use inside and outside the hospital; a receptacle permitting use of conventional electrocardiographic electrodes to transmit the cardiac rhythm to the oscilloscope; and an output jack for connection to the electrocardiogram so that cardiac rhythm can be recorded upon a strip chart if desired. A separate synchronizing system can be bought for elective cardioversion. This extremely practical monitor-defibrillator unit can be taken anywhere inside or outside the cardiac receiving room and can be used for prehospital cardiac care by a cardiac ambulance team, for in-hospital mobile coronary care to transport patients from the emergency department to the coronary care or intensive care units, and for the hospital cardiac arrest team.

If the emergency department is a particularly active one, it may be desirable to equip several observation and treatment rooms with cardiac defibrillators. An inexpensive AC-powered cardiac defibrillator made by Physio Control delivers unsynchronized direct current shocks up to 400 watt-seconds (Fig. 38). These defibrillators may be used to supplement the most essential equipment described earlier, are useful in the management of sudden ventricular fibrillation but are incapable of detecting and monitoring, and must be plugged into an AC wall receptacle to function.

A number of manufacturers offer battery-powered electrocardiographic recorders. Small, light, rugged units are preferable because they may be used anywhere, and there is no need to waste time searching for an AC wall receptacle when confronting a cardiac emergency. The electrocardiogram should be equipped with circuitry to protect it against large surges of electrical energy such as the direct current shock of cardiac defibrillation. Electrocardiographic recorders powered by AC

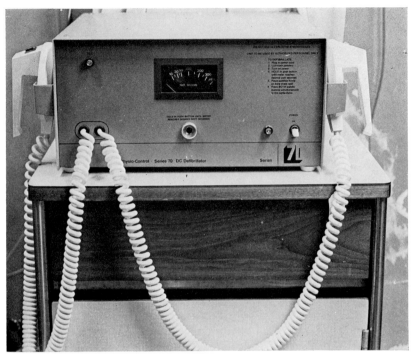

Figure 38. This inexpensive unsynchronized AC-powered cardiac defibrillator may supplement the more sophisticated battery-powered equipment. Its long cables easily allow use between two cardiac beds.

current should be grounded and also have protective circuitry against the current surge of cardiac defibrillation.

The battery-powered external fixed-rate cardiac pacemaker is useful until a temporary transvenous demand-pacing system is established. The Electrodyne TR-3 (Westwood, Massachusetts) unit is satisfactory for urgent external cardiac pacing and may be used temporarily as an internal pacemaker. For sudden asystole, when fist pacing does not work, a number 18 cardiac needle can be quickly inserted through the fourth or fifth intercostal space into the right ventricle, and a pacing electrode may be quickly introduced (Electro-Catheter, Rahway, New Jersey). Pacing can be accomplished in this situation using the Electrodyne unit, but it is preferable to use a demand-pacing unit if competitive ventricular dysrhythmias occur. The Medtronic 5880 (Minneapolis, Minnesota) battery-powered external pacemaker, which has both demand and fixed modes for pacing, is an ideal unit once an intracardiac electrode has been positioned properly.

In the management of sudden, unexpected cardiopulmonary arrest, it is essential to have suction available to clear away oropharyngeal and tracheal secretions and to have oxygen to administer during assisted ventilation. In the emergency department, suction and oxygen can be provided from outlets on the walls. When building a new emergency department or updating an old one, it is often possible to establish a central hospital source for suction and for oxygen, with outlets for both in the observation and treatment rooms of the emergency department. This assures permanent sources for suction and delivery of oxygen. If wall suction is not available, a battery-powered (Laerdal, Tuckahoe, New York) or AC-powered (Gomco, Buffalo, New York) suction pump must be kept in the cardiac receiving room. For operation outside the hospital or in the hospital where wall receptacles are not immediately available, the battery-powered Laerdal suction pump will function for thirty minutes before discharging its battery.

The needs of the small hospital's cardiac receiving room can be met by a battery-powered monitor-defibrillator, battery-powered external cardiac pacemaker, battery-powered electrocardiographic recorder, and battery-powered suction machine, which allow movement of equipment from room to room or on the stretcher with the patient and are versatile and safe. Where possible, the cardiac receiving room should also have its own permanent cardiac monitoring system with an oscilloscope containing a five-inch screen for each patient, an audible beep signal for cardiac rhythm, and an alarm system triggered by low and high levels of heart rate (Fig. 39). This system is powered by conventional AC wall receptacles, and a slave oscilloscope should be available in the central nurses' station of the emergency department so that the charge nurse may observe the rhythm in case the patient is unexpectedly left alone in the cardiac receiving room. Continuous observation of the oscilloscopic screen is most desirable but frequently not possi-

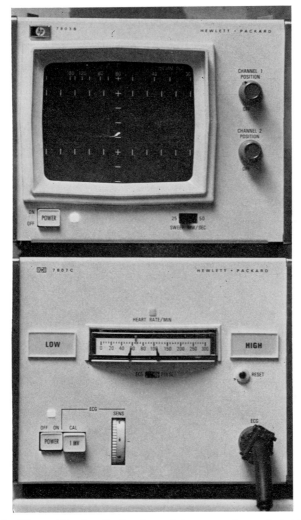

Figure 39. These Hewlett-Packard modules provide a bedside look at heart rate and rhythm and may be connected to a beeper, slave oscilloscope, and alarm outside the cardiac receiving room.

ble because of a shortage of personnel in the emergency department or hospital. The beep signal provides another way of alerting the staff that a dysrhythmia is present and is particularly valuable, since clinically significant dysrhythmias such as ventricular premature beats may occur within the limits set for the heart rate alarm. Slowing or acceleration of the heart rate beyond the limits set by the staff, usually below 60 or above 110 beats/min, will trigger the heart-rate alarm. Staff must be available to observe the cardiac rhythm on the oscilloscope, to hear the rhythm of the beep signal, and to respond to the heart-rate alarm. An intercom system is necessary so that help can be obtained quickly without abandoning the patient even temporarily.

All hospitals should have a standard emergency drug box and emergency ventilating tray for use in dealing with sudden cardiopulmonary arrest.[3] These modules should be provided by the hospital pharmacy and central supply. Each box should have a permanent external list of its contents and a seal which if broken requires the hospital staff to return the module for inspection and restocking by the pharmacy or by hospital central supply. The emergency drug box and emergency ventilating tray should be kept on the crash cart of the emergency department and on an open shelf in the cardiac receiving room. Table I lists the medications kept in the emergency drug box at the University of Virginia Medical Center and Table II lists the contents of the emergency ventilating tray.

All the battery-powered equipment described is adequate for dealing with cardiac emergencies in the prehospital phase and in the cardiac receiving room. This equipment is also suitable for the conduct of in-hospital mobile coronary care and for stocking the crash cart of the hospital cardiac arrest team. In small community hospitals, the cardiac arrest crash cart may respond from the emergency department or from the coronary care or intensive care units. It is vitally important that the cardiac emergency equipment and medications remain easily accessible for use when needed for the diagnosis and management of sudden cardiopulmonary arrest. Therefore, this equipment and the medications should always be left in an easily visible, central location and never be locked in a closet or stored in such a manner as to prevent its prompt use in the care of a patient.

If the emergency department is viewed in the larger context of a critical care complex, one may need a larger number of cardiac observation units. For example, the cardiac receiving

TABLE I
CONTENTS OF CARDIAC EMERGENCY DRUG BOX

Drugs	Quantity
Aminophylline 500 mg/20 ml I.V.	2 ampuls
Atropine sulfate 0.4 mg/1 ml 20 ml	1 vial
Calcium chloride 1 gm/10 ml	2 ampuls
Digoxin (Lanoxin) 0.5 mg/2 ml	2 ampuls
Diphenhydramine (Benadryl) 50 mg/1 ml	2 ampuls
Epinephrine 1:10,000 10 ml	2 ampuls
Furosemide (Lasix) 20 mg/2 ml	2 ampuls
Hydrocortisone (Solu-Cortef) 100 mg	4 vials
Isoproterenol (Isuprel) 1 mg/5 ml	6 ampuls
Lidocaine (Xylocaine) 20 mg/1 ml 5 ml	4 ampuls
Lidocaine (Xylocaine) 20 mg/1 ml 50 ml	2 ampuls
Metaraminol (Aramine) 10 mg/1 ml 10 ml	1 vial
Norepinephrine (Levophed) 0.2% 4 ml	6 ampuls
Normal saline 30 ml	1 vial
Levallorphan (Lorfan) 1 mg/1 ml	1 ampul
Phenylephrine (Neosynephrine) 10 mg/1 ml 5 ml	1 vial
Phenobarbital (Luminal) 130 mg/1 ml	2 ampuls
Potassium chloride 2 mEq/ml 30 ml	2 vials
Reserpine (Serpasil) 5 mg/12 ml	1 ampul
Sodium bicarbonate 44.6 mEq (isoject)	8 ampuls
Equipment	
Ampul files	2
Needles	
#19	6
#20	6
#21	2
#25	2
Syringes	
2 cc	3
5 cc	3
10 cc	3
Tourniquet	1
Alcohol swabs	10
Heart needles	
#18	2
#20	2

Supplies Outside Drug Box on Crash Cart	
Dextrose 5% 500 cc	1 bottle
Dextrose 5% in normal saline 500 cc	1 bottle
Normal saline 500 cc	1 bottle
Intravenous tubing set	2
Intravenous tubing extension sets	2
Stopcock	1

room might be equipped with two to four beds, each with its own electrocardiographic monitoring and alarm system with a slave oscilloscope observable at the emergency department's central nurses station. A single cardiac defibrillator might serve this four-patient unit. If the volume of cardiac emergencies treated by the hospital emergency department justifies this size of cardiac receiving room, this area would provide a safe

TABLE II

CARDIAC EMERGENCY VENTILATING TRAY

1 Laryngoscope handle (batteries and bulbs)
1 Adult blade #3
1 Child's blade #2
1 Infant's blade #1
1 Mask casting
1 Oxygen needle valve regulator connected with oxygen tubing with
        plastic needle connectors
1 Breathing bag
1 Adult face mask
1 Child's face mask
1 Copper Stylette (with guard)
1 Adult Resusitube
1 Infant Resusitube
1 Airway #5
1 Airway #3
1 Airway #2
1 Suction catheter #14
1 Suction catheter #10
1 12 cc Syringe (disposable)
1 Blunt needle #18
1 Catheter adapter (Christmas Tree)
1 Hemostat
1 Tube surgical lubricant (water soluble)
1 Tongue depressor
Endotracheal tubes:
        1 #2 13.5 cm with 4 mm connector
        1 #4 17.0 cm with 4 mm connector
        1 #6 19.0 cm with 6 mm connector
        1 #7 19.0 cm with 7 mm connector (cuffed)
        1 #8 20.0 cm with 8 mm conne_tor (cuffed)
        1 #16 Coles with 4 mm connector
        1 #9 22.0 cm with 9 mm connector (cuffed)

Note: The oxygen needle valve, oxygen tubing, plastic connector, breathing bag, mask
    casting, and adult mask should be assembled and ready to use. The syringe
    should be assembled with either the blunt needle or catheter adapter attached
    to it.

environment for the diagnosis and treatment of cardiac emergencies. In large metropolitan hospitals, it is sometimes possible to create the ideal critical care complex in which the cardiac, medical, and surgical intensive care units are located next to or as a part of the emergency department. Skilled personnel and all necessary equipment are instantly available to the patient from the moment of entry into such an emergency department.

POLICY AND PRACTICE

The cardiac receiving room must provide personnel, medications, and equipment, not only to diagnose and treat cardiac arrest with efficient cardiopulmonary resuscitation but also provide precoronary care with close observation and treatment, thereby preventing the need for resuscitation. The cardiac receiving room should become the safest holding area for patients awaiting entry to the hospital coronary care unit or intensive care unit rather than the conventional admitting office. It is particularly important that cardiac patients not wait in physicians' offices or in elective hospital admitting areas where detection of life-threatening dysrhythmias and cardiac arrest is left to chance and where cardiac arrest cannot be managed easily. Physicians requesting admission for cardiac patients should direct these patients through the hospital emergency department via the cardiac receiving room rather than through the hospital admitting office if a bed is not immediately available in the coronary care or intensive care units.

Initial and urgent cardiac evaluation and treatment are always carried out in the cardiac receiving room. Far more important than racks of expensive equipment is the intelligent observation and treatment of cardiac patients. When a patient enters the cardiac receiving room, the nurse records the pulse, respirations, and blood pressure, places electrocardiographic electrodes on the patient, and records a twelve-lead electrocardiogram. If dysrhythmias predisposing to ventricular fibrillation or to asystole are noted, the nurse and medical staff must be prepared to treat with appropriate medications and external cardiac pacing. If the patient suddenly becomes apneic, pulseless, and cyanotic, ventilation and external cardiac massage must be started right away and additional help summoned using an intercom system. Cardiac defibrillation should be attempted immediately since ventricular fibrillation has a good prognosis when promptly removed.[10] Heart-lung resuscitative measures should be carried on until blood pressure, pulse, and respirations are adequate. An easily palpable femoral or carotid pulse is good evidence of restoration of cardiac function. Ventilation should be continued until adequate spontaneous respiratory tidal volume is clinically apparent and cyanosis has disappeared.

IN-HOSPITAL MOBILE CORONARY CARE

When the patient's cardiac problem has been clarified, his general condition and cardiac rhythm have stabilized under treatment, and his transportation to the coronary care or intensive care units can be considered safe, the in-hospital mobile coronary care unit should be used to transfer the patient from the cardiac receiving room to the coronary care or intensive care units. In its simplest form, in-hospital mobile coronary care means transporting the patient with a nurse or physician in attendance trained to monitor the cardiac rhythm, to administer medications for dysrhythmias, to use the external cardiac pacemaker, and to perform cardiac defibrillation. Freshly prepared syringes of lidocaine and atropine can be taped to the case of the defibrillator and can be given intravenously if needed during the patient's journey from the cardiac receiving room to the coronary care unit. When it is necessary to admit a patient for acute cardiac care, the coronary care or intensive care unit is notified. The coronary care nursing and medical staff may come down to transport the patient with a battery-powered monitor-defibrillator, or alternatively, members of the nursing and physician staff of the emergency department may transport the patient to the coronary care unit. Thus, once intensive cardiac care conditions have been established in the cardiac receiving room, these intensive care conditions hopefully are never disrupted until the patient is under electrocardiographic observation in the coronary care or intensive care unit.[11] During use of this type of in-hospital mobile coronary care unit to transport over 1000 acutely ill cardiac patients, there has not been a cardiac arrest.[12]

NURSE AND PHYSICIAN STAFFING

Staffing the cardiac receiving room will depend upon the number of doctors and nurses available to the emergency department, hospital, and community. In a large hospital medical center, the emergency department has at least one resident physician in constant attendance who takes his meals in the area and sleeps in a call room built into the emergency department. Nursing staff is always present. Hence management of the patient in the cardiac receiving room is facilitated by the constant presence of trained personnel. However, in other hospitals, the resident physician may be always present in the building but may eat, sleep, and perform duties elsewhere as well as attending to patients in the cardiac receiving room upon request. Some hospitals without resident medical staff employ physicians to work full-time in the emergency department. In communities with fewer physicians, the doctor may be present in the hospital all day long and during incidental evening and night hours when he is visiting patients. However, in such a community, the physician may not always be present in the hospital, and the nurse becomes the resident medical staff in terms of emergency service to cardiac patients. Where medical manpower is even thinner, the physician may be present in the hospital for only parts of the day, evening, or night, reflecting his obligations to hospital and nonhospital patients. In this situation, the nurse also acts as the medical staff of the cardiac receiving room.

In the community hospital, two possibilities for nurses to staff the emergency department and cardiac receiving room exist. In hospitals with adequate nursing staff, a nurse may always attend the emergency department and be available to care for the patient in the cardiac receiving room. In hospitals in smaller communities or where inadequate numbers of nurses are available, the nurse may serve in another part of the hospital and respond on call to the emergency department for patients with acute cardiac problems. In this latter situation, the emergency department receptionist represents the first individual to confront cardiac and other emergencies. Obviously, it is undesirable to have a completely untrained individual as the first line of defense in dealing with cardiac emergencies. Therefore, the most skilled nurses in the community hospital, such as the nurse specialist in cardiology or intensive coronary care, should come to the cardiac receiving room to care for the patient with a suspected heart attack, to begin an intravenous drip, to initiate monitoring, to relieve pain and stabilize dysrhythmias, and to transport the patient using a monitor-defibrillator to the coronary care or intensive care area. This type of cardiac nursing practice has been very successful at the Anne Arundel Community Hospital, Annapolis, Maryland.[13]

For nurses to function adequately in the cardiac receiving room, they must be well educated in cardiopulmonary resuscitation, cardiac defibrillation, external cardiac pacing, and administration of medications to prevent the need for resuscitation by controlling dysrhythmias. If the staff nurse in the emergency department cannot provide these services, a nurse trained in intensive or coronary care should be available on call to the emergency department. In a community hospital with a large volume of cardiac emergencies, it is well worthwhile providing the emergency department nurse with the same special training as the coronary care or intensive care nurse. Indeed, after completion of a course in critical cardiac care, the emergency department nurse should periodically recycle through the coronary care or intensive care unit for a practical refresher course.

PREHOSPITAL CARE OF CARDIAC EMERGENCIES

Facilities and Personnel

Coronary accidents are among the leading causes of death outside the hospital in the United States. In the past decade much has been learned about diagnosing and treating acute coronary accidents and in many instances disability and death can be prevented or delayed by application of available medical skills and knowledge.[1,2] A community organizing itself to provide care for cardiac emergencies should create or combine an existing hospital emergency department and coronary care unit, ambulance system, and emergency personnel structure with the most portable and practical equipment presently available for cardiac intensive care. This overall organization should include professional and volunteer ambulance and rescue workers educated in the care of the patient with a cardiac crisis, an adequate number of battery-powered monitor-defibrillator, external pacemaker and electrocardiographic recorder units, and an emergency telephone information center in which the ambulance service or rescue squad share an emergency telephone line with the emergency department and hospital coronary care unit.[4] Since most rescue squads and ambulance services have shortwave radio equipment, it is possible to include transmission of electrocardiograms and a central transmitting and receiving cardiac station located in the coronary care unit or emergency department of the hospital to serve those patients outside the hospital at various levels of approach to hospital cardiac care.[14,15]

A mobile cardiac intensive care unit or cardiac ambulance responding to emergency calls can best provide facilities of hospital intensive care and skilled personnel who can render

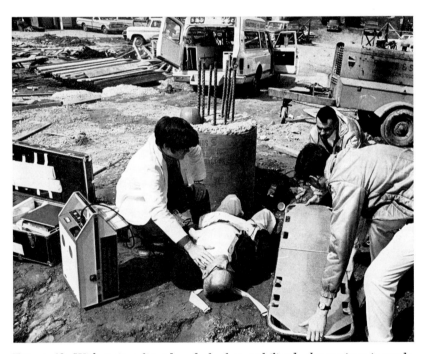

Figure 40. With pain relieved and rhythm stabilized, the patient is ready to be transported directly to the hospital coronary care unit, bypassing the emergency department. Note the electrode cable between the patient and the monitor-defibrillator for continous observation of cardiac rhythm, and the standard ambulance in the background. No speed and no sirens are needed while returning to the hospital, since the patient has been in an intensive care unit since arrival of cardiac ambulance team. (Courtesy of the *Charlottesville Daily Progress*.)

cardiac first aid, thus preventing disability and death from coronary disease.[1,5,6,7,16,17] The ideal cardiac ambulance team is composed of a physician, nurse, and two rescue workers or emergency medical technicians. Frequently, it is not possible to provide this concentration of medical manpower, and the nurse or physician may function in each other's absence with the rescue workers. A redistribution of priorities is necessary on the part of the nursing and medical profession in order to meet the needs of the patient with a cardiac emergency outside the hospital.

A model of cardiac ambulance service for small communities can easily be developed through cooperation amongst the physicians, nurses, and rescue squad or ambulance service. The minimum equipment needed costs less than $5000 (Fig. 41), and no special ambulance is necessary, although it is much easier to work with cardiac patients in an ambulance with at least five feet of overhead room between the floor and ceiling. In larger or wealthy communities, a special cardiac ambulance can be constructed which is virtually a mobile intensive cardiac care unit with over six feet of inside head room. It should be emphasized that such ambulances are a luxury, and many communities which can not afford expensive equipment can provide adequate cardiac intensive care facilities in their existing ambulance systems.[1,6,16,17]

In practice, the physician often clearly identifies a cardiac emergency over the phone and activates the rescue squad or ambulance service. If the physician is nearby, the ambulance could conveniently take the physician and the equipment and medications for cardiac care to the patient. Alternatively, the ambulance could pick up an appropriately trained nurse and the equipment and medications from the emergency department of the community hospital. For rapid service, the ambulance may be stocked with the conventional battery-powered equipment for cardiac diagnosis and intensive care and a supply of the appropriate emergency medications. However, in many communities, a single ambulance cannot be reserved for cardiac emergencies. In this situation, it is best to have the depot of equipment in the cardiac receiving room of the emer-

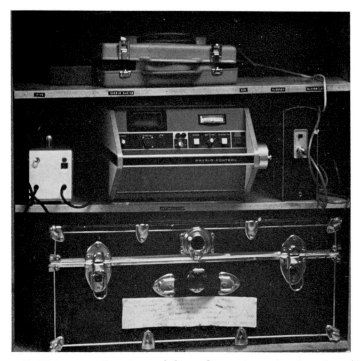

Figure 41. This comprehensive mobile cardiac unit costing less than $5000 provides prehospital cardiac care. The same equipment is useful inside the hospital (see text for details). On the top shelf, the suction pump is charging. On the middle shelf, the quick-charger (left), the monitor-defibrillator (center), and the electrocardiograph (right) are seen. On the bottom shelf, the footlocker contains the external pacemaker and the medications listed in Tables I, II, and III. When activated for a cardiac emergency, the suction pump and the electrocardiograph are placed in the locker. During charging, heat generated makes it advisable to keep the suction pump and the electrocardiograph outside the locker.

gency department of the hospital located nearest the ambulance service or rescue squad headquarters (Fig. 41).

The creation of an emergency telephone information center is advisable, since a call directly to the rescue squad or ambulance service may require screening by hospital personnel.[4] A common telephone line connecting the ambulance dispatcher, emergency department, coronary care unit, and doctor's office and home provides rapid communication amongst the patient and cardiac emergency personnel. Emergency calls suggestive of heart attack coming to the rescue squad or ambulance service may be screened by the dispatcher briefly or passed directly on to a nurse or doctor in the emergency department, hospital coronary care unit, office, or home. If activated, the ambulance team could pick up the nurse or doctor on the way to the patient in distress. Ideally, the rescue squad headquarters or ambulance depot should be built within the hospital complex or very close by. This proximity of emergency ambulance service and hospital would allow for quick addition of the nurse or doctor for cardiac emergency trips. Equally important, proximity would provide the time and opportunity for volunteer rescue or salaried ambulance workers to maintain or expand their skills by working under the supervision of the physician and nurse with patients in the emergency department, intensive care unit, or coronary care unit. Thus, rescue and ambulance workers would be involved continuously in work that maintained or improved their skills in caring for patients with critical illnesses, including cardiac emergencies.

Cardiac ambulance service might also be carried out, as in a number of communities already, by nurses or trained cardiac ambulance workers who maintain radio contact with a physician or nurse in the hospital coronary care unit. This type of cardiac emergency service provides legal protection for the nurse or ambulance worker, since the diagnosis is established and the treatment is carried out with voice contact between the physician and the nurse or cardiac ambulance worker. Furthermore, the electrocardiogram can be transmitted via radio or telephone to the physician for diagnosis. The conversation between the ambulance personnel and the physician and the electrocardiogram can conveniently be recorded, thus providing documentation of the cardiac emergency call.[14,15]

In providing improved care for patients with a cardiac emergency, serious consideration should be given to making better use of existing ambulance systems. For example, in New Jersey there are over 400 squads of volunteer rescue workers, and in Virginia there are 165 rescue squads. Since these groups of rescue workers have demonstrated considerable aptitude in learning techniques such as cardiopulmonary resuscitation, they should be educated further in the diagnosis and management of cardiac emergencies and about the use of portable equipment, medications, and special procedures such as cardiac defibrillation and external cardiac pacing. Salaried specialists in emergency care in police and fire departments of a number of cities have been trained to provide superb care for cardiac emergencies. Legislation in Florida and Washington has recognized the function of well-trained emergency medical technicians in providing comprehensive cardiac first aid, including defibrillation and administration of drugs.

Equipment and Medications

The cardiac emergency drug box (Table I) and ventilating tray (Table II) used in prehospital coronary care are identical to that used in the cardiac receiving room and throughout the general hospital. All of the equipment and medications for prehospital coronary care, except for the monitor-defibrillator, are kept in a footlocker. The contents are checked and the electrocardiogram, suction machine, and monitor-defibrillator are set in the recharging mode to replenish their depleted batteries after each response to a call from the community (Fig. 41). Table III lists the equipment and medications needed for prehospital cardiac emergencies. The only supplies outside the footlocker consist of four drugs in freshly prepared syringes changed daily. Morphine, pentazocine, lidocaine, and atropine are refrigerated and kept in a small case with a tourniquet and alcohol sponges ready for instant use. The monitor-defibrillator constitutes a separate burden, but the footlocker, defibrillator, and small drug case are easily carried by two persons.

Policy and Practice

Emergency calls suggestive of heart attack coming to the physician are screened, and the cardiac ambulance is activated. Cardiac calls coming directly to the ambulance dispatcher may be briefly screened by the dispatcher or referred to the staff of

TABLE III
EQUIPMENT AND DRUGS FOR
PREHOSPITAL CARDIAC EMERGENCIES

Contents of Locker

1 Battery-powered suction machine (Laerdal)
1 Battery-powered electrocardiogram (Physio Control)
1 External pacemaker (Electrodyne)
1 ECG patch cable (from defibrillator to ECG)
1 Set of ECG electrodes
1 Emergency drug box (contents in Table I)
1 Emergency ventilating box (contents in Table II)
Intravenous solutions
    1 - 500 cc dextrose 5%
    1 - 500 cc dextrose 5% in normal saline
1 Emesis basin
Arm boards
    2 Short
    2 Long
2 ECG strip chart rolls
5 Penrose drains for use as tourniquets for pulmonary edema
1 Blood pressure cuff
1 Stethoscope
2 Tongue blades
1 Scissors
4 Towels
Intravenous kit
    3 Micro drips
    Tourniquet
    Antibiotic ointment (Neosporin)
    2 #18 longdwell
    2 #19 scalp vein
    2 #21 scalp vein
    4 - 50 cc syringe
    3 - 12 cc syringe
    3 - 6 cc syringe
    4 - 3½ cc syringe
History and physical forms, tablet of each
Mobile coronary care unit log book

Supplies outside locker

In a small case, 2 syringes of each medication are drawn up ready for use.
    Morphine
    Pentazocine
    Lidocaine
    Atropine
Monitor-defibrillator (Physio Control)

the emergency department or coronary care unit. A screening questionnaire is helpful for the ambulance dispatcher and for the staff of the emergency department and coronary care unit. The name, location, sex, age, and telephone number of the patient should be quickly recorded. In general, a heart attack is unusual in a man under 25 or a woman under 45, and screening the complaint of younger individuals should be passed on to the hospital staff. However, the well-trained ambulance dispatcher may obtain positive responses about chest pain, breathlessness, sweating, previous heart attack, fainting or collapse, radiation of pain, and quality of pain, and activate the cardiac ambulance. When the ambulance dispatcher contacts the hospital emergency department or coronary care unit, he continues to listen in to the conference between the patient and the hospital staff for educational as well as service purposes.

Cardiac first aid can be quickly provided in a number of ways, depending upon the size of the community, traffic pattern, and number and type of personnel and ambulances. When activated, the cardiac ambulance may proceed to the hospital emergency department or physician's office or home to collect medical personnel, medications, and equipment and then go to the patient. Where personnel and ambulances are plentiful, one ambulance team may go directly to the patient, and a second ambulance may bring the physician or nurse a few minutes later. If an ambulance team confronts a previously unidentified cardiac emergency, they may summon the cardiac ambulance by radio.

At the scene of the cardiac emergency, the rescue workers place the monitor paddles of the monitor-defibrillator upon the chest so that the cardiac rhythm can be observed immediately (Fig. 37). Electrocardiographic telemetry and voice radio communication simultaneously may be carried out with hospital staff in the emergency department or coronary care unit[14,15] (Biocom, Culver City, California; Pioneer Medical Systems, New Britain, Connecticut). An intravenous drip is started for ease of administering medications. Under remote[14,15] or direct supervision, appropriate medications are given to relieve pain and stabilize cardiac rhythm.[1,2,3] A twelve-lead electrocardiogram may be obtained using a battery-powered recorder. Once the patient's condition has stabilized, it is safe to place the patient on a stretcher (Fig. 40), while conducting continuous monitoring, and return to the hospital without the use of speed or sirens.[1] If difficulties arise during transport, the ambulance is stopped, and all cardiac ambulance personnel join in treating the patient until his condition is restabilized. Then the journey back to the hospital is resumed. Upon arrival at the hospital, the cardiac patient is moved directly into the coronary care or intensive care unit without stopping in the cardiac receiving room of the emergency department.[1] Only if the patient has clearly not had a cardiac disturbance may he be left in the emergency department for further evaluation.

Nurses, physicians, rescue workers, and ambulance technicians may remain on call for emergency service to the out-of-the-hospital cardiac patient while working at many useful regular duties, provided temporary backup staff is available when they are out on a cardiac ambulance call. In general, trips to care for patients vary from 20 to 60 minutes, but average about 40 minutes away from the hospital. The number of such cardiac episodes removing nursing or physician personnel from the hospital will vary with the size of the population served and the type of community. Obviously, education of the community, its physicians and nurses, and its rescue and ambulance workers to make use of the cardiac ambulance system will make greater demands upon the ambulance team as goes on.

Metropolitan and suburban cardiac ambulance services have proved practicable in Belfast, Ireland;[1,16] New York City;[6] Jacksonville and Miami, Florida; Seattle, Washington; Portland, Oregon; Columbus, Ohio; Montgomery County, Maryland; Newark, New Jersey; and Los Angeles and San Francisco, California. Rural cardiac ambulances function in Ballymena, Ireland,[5] and in Pennsylvania; North Carolina; and Charlottesville, Virginia.[17] Thus, the cardiac receiving room and emergency department can extend into the community to care specifically for the cardiac patient when he is at highest risk from sudden death.[1]

REFERENCES

1. Pantridge, J.F.: Mobile coronary care. *Chest*, 58:229, 1970.
2. Lown, B., Klein, M.D., and Hershberg, P.I.: Coronary and precoronary care. *Am J Med*, 46:705, 1969.
3. Grace, W.J.: *Coronary Care Unit.* New York, Appleton-Century-Crofts, 1970.
4. Yu, P.N., Bielski, M.T., Edwards, A., Friedberg, C.K., Grace, W.J.,

January, L.E., Likoff, W., Scherlis, L., and Weissler, A.M.: Resources for the optimal care of patients with acute myocardial infarction. *Circulation, 43:*A-171, 1971.

5. Kernohan, R.J., and McGucken, R.B.: Mobile intensive care in myocardial infarction. *Br Med J, 3:*178, 1968.

6. Grace, W.J., and Chadbourn, J.A.: The mobile coronary care unit. *Dis Chest, 55:*452, 1969.

7. Grace, W.J.: The mobile coronary care unit and the intermediate coronary care unit in the total systems approach to acute myocardial infarction. *Chest, 58:*363, 1970.

8. Starmer, C.F., McIntosh, H.D., and Whalen, R.E.: Electrical hazards and cardiovascular function. *N Eng J Med, 284:*181, 1971.

9. Adgey, A.A.J., Scott, M.E., Allen, J.D., Nelson, P.G., Geddes, J.S., Zaidi, S.A., and Pantridge, J.F.: Management of ventricular fibrillation outside hospital. *Lancet, 1:*1169, 1969.

10. McNamee, B.T., Robinson, T.J., Adgey, A.A.J., Scott, M.E., Geddes, J.S., and Pantridge, J.F.: Long-term prognosis following ventricular fibrillation in acute ischemic heart disease. *Br Med J, 4:*204, 1970.

11. Taylor, J.O., Landers, C.F., Chulay, J.D., Hood, W.B., Jr., and Abelmann, W.H.: Monitoring high-risk cardiac patients during transportation in hospital. *Lancet, 2:*1205, 1970.

12. Crampton, R.S.: Mobile coronary care in hospital. *Lancet, 1:*296, 1971.

13. Church, G., and Biern, R.O.: Intensive coronary care—a practical system for a small hospital without house staff. *N Eng J Med, 281:*1155, 1969.

14. Woodwark, G.M., and Gillespie, I.A.: Monitoring of ambulance patients by radio telemetry. *Can Med Assoc J, 102:*1277, 1970.

15. Nagel, E.L., Hirschman, J.C., Nussenfeld, S.R., Rankin, D., and Lundblad, E.: Telemetry—medical command in coronary and other mobile emergency care systems. *JAMA, 214:*332, 1970.

16. Barker, J.M., Chaturvedi, N.C., Groves, D.H.M., Shivalingappa, G., Boyle, D.McC., Gamble, J., Millar, D.S., Walsh, M.J., and Wilson, H.K.: Mobile coronary care. *Lancet, 2:*133, 1970.

17. Crampton, R.S., and Herndon, N.C., Jr.: Heart attack rescue service. *First Aid Bull Virginia Assoc Vol Rescue Squads, 28:*6, 1971.

II. NONCARDIAC MEDICAL EMERGENCIES

WILLIAM E. HOOPER

The preparation for and care of minor medical emergencies seldom requires more experience and skills than those possessed by the average physician. Neither do they require more equipment than he is likely to carry in his "little black bag." The discussion here will center on more serious and complex medical emergencies that do require extra skills and extra equipment, and particularly their preemergency mobilization. The title of a recent review of emergency room care, *Hurry up—but think*[1] might be a good motto to follow.

Many noncardiac emergencies commonly require a rapid institution of life-sustaining procedures, along with the simultaneous evaluation of the patient's pathophysiological condition. The medical emergency is one of the most frequent-occurring happenings in the emergency department, challenging the physician's total skills. The physician, by prompt and efficient management, can appreciably reduce morbidity and mortality here more often than in any other area of medical practice. He must manage the patient with alacrity rather than haste, must know the *do nots* as well as the *dos*, and must perform what is required only and not be guilty of blind assumptions that lead only to unnecessary and complicating procedures. The medical emergency is a definite time of stress both for patient and physician. However, it is only the physician who can resolve the problem.

Although we will consider the management of the comatose patient as he typically arrives at an emergency department, his management is applicable to all noncardiac medical emergencies regardless of the level of consciousness. An attempt will be made to outline a procedure (not fixed or routine) for the care of the patient in that most vital first 60 minutes. The initial problem is the sustaining and supporting of the essential

268

dynamics of life while in search for a diagnosis. In the majority of cases, he may be required to work without an adequate or even helpful history. With a comatose patient, the evaluation and initial treatment must proceed simultaneously without the advantage of a working diagnosis. Therefore, the problem is reduced to sustaining life until a specific diagnosis can be ascertained and definite appropriate treatment instituted.

POSITIONING AND INITIAL PREPARATION

On arrival, the patient is placed in the supine position on a firm table or stretcher that can provide for orthopneic positioning. (See illustrations of stretchers in Chapter 5 on equipment.) The room must be well lighted and have within it the necessary equipment for emergency procedures. There must be adequate clearance around the table for freedom of movement by the physicians, nurses, and paramedical personnel. Clutter must be avoided, as it breeds confusion. (The necessity for adequate working space is discussed in detail in Chapter 3 on plans and planning—JHS.) The patient's clothing must be removed. The prime factors in the initiation of management are the establishment of an airway, evaluation of ventilation, securing a route for intravenous fluids, obtaining blood specimens, evaluation of pulse and blood pressure, and control of any hemorrhage.

VENTILATION

This necessitates airway patency and adequate pulmonary oxygen exchange, along with adequate circulation. The most common ventilation problem is the obstruction of upper respiratory passages. The importance and simplicity of establishing an airway cannot be overemphasized. These obstructions can be easily corrected by forefinger scanning of the patient's mouth and pharynx. The patient is kept in the supine position, the chin is elevated, and the neck extended. Any foreign bodies, including dentures, are removed and an oral pharyngeal airway inserted. Suction must be employed to remove any secretions, blood, or mucus. The oral pharyngeal airway must be of proper size and be placed over and behind the tongue. If the patient is not breathing on his own, mouth-to-mouth breathing or squeeze-bag positive-pressure inflation is the next step. This assist can be used with or without oxygen. The Ambu bag mask is commonly used today and has the advantage of allowing the physician to observe the patient while administering the ventilating assist. (This and other models are illustrated in Chapter 5 on equipment.) Awareness of the danger of tracheal bronchial obstruction is important, and oscillation of the chest to evaluate insuflation is a simple but useful mechanism.

If by these measures, adequate respiratory control is not obtained, one must consider an endotracheal tube. The indications for intubation are the unconscious patient requiring assisted ventilation, inadequacy of the oral pharyngeal airway to maintain a patent airway, threatening aspiration of stomach contents, inadequate spontaneous clearing of the tracheal bronchial secretions, and/or anticipation of a tracheostomy. An endotracheal tube is preferable to a tracheostomy and has the advantage of being less traumatic as well as a more rapid procedure. Emergency department personnel should be trained in this procedure. The intubation can prevent brain damage from hypoxia when instituted early enough. Supplemental oxygen, when given, should be limited to 30 to 40 percent concentration. A Ventimask® controls the concentration on the basis of the venturi principle, by admixing 100 percent oxygen and ambient air. A patient on oxygen must be watched for respiratory distress by observing the level of consciousness, respiratory rate, and frequent measurements of arterial pCO_2. The interpretation of blood gases can be simplified by using a 50–50 rule. If the pCO_2 is greater than 50 mm Hg and the pO_2 is less than 50 mm Hg, supplemental oxygen is required. Treatment cannot be delayed while getting blood gas readings. Action must precede diagnosis with any respiratory problem.

CIRCULATION

When the pulmonary phase of tissue oxygenation has been established, the circulatory system must be evaluated and corrective measures instituted to insure perfusion. Although we have considered ventilation first, while the procedures to establish adequate ventilation are occurring, another physician or nurse should be checking the pulse and blood pressure and recording them by time and establishing an intravenous fluid route. An 18-gauge needle or large intracatheter is inserted, and when the veins are poor, a cut down must be performed. Once this is accomplished, enough blood can be obtained for stat or delayed studies. The vital signs should be recorded when obtained and the time noted each time they are recorded. The changes in these over a period of time may be as important as the readings themselves. When checking pulse rate, rhythm, and character, always include precordial, femoral, and carotid as well as radial pulses. If the rate exceeds 180 per minute or is irregular, the possibility of pulmonary edema and vascular collapse is enhanced. Systolic blood pressures of less than 90 mm Hg endanger cerebral perfusion. If this is the case and the intravenous fluid is not evoking response, the insertion of a central venous pressure apparatus is indicated. The possibility of shock in a medical emergency must always be considered. The CVP (central venous pressure) is the most reliable procedure in the diagnosis and treatment of shock. Low CVP readings indicate an absolute or relative hypovolemia and the need to expand the intravascular volume. High CVP readings are present in inadequate cardiac output and circulation overload. There are no contraindications to employing the CVP route for the administration of fluids. With low CVP readings, vaso pressure drugs as well as blood plasma and isotonic saline and occasionally Dextran must be considered. The danger of overloading the circulatory system as long as the CVP remains below 150 millimeters of saline is unlikely.

HISTORY

An attempt to gather any pertinent features of the patient's history must be made, with emphasis on previous hospital admissions, previous illnesses, medications, injury, drug ingestion, and environment. Relatives, friends, police, or anyone else escorting the patient to the hospital must be detained for questioning. A search of the patient's personal effects for information or for telephone numbers frequently results in obtaining supplemental information. It proves best for one of the nursing staff to initiate the fact finding until the emergency physician has time to begin this phase.

PHYSICAL FINDINGS AND EVALUATION

Even though we are considering noncardiac medical emergencies, a total body check for evidence of trauma or internal or external bleeding must not be omitted. A search for bites and needle punctures must be accomplished. The skin is checked for moisture, texture, and pallor. Temperature is recorded. The level of consciousness, response to painful stimuli, limb movement, and evidence of lateralizing signs are all observed in the initial body scan. The head is examined for any evidence of facial asymmetry, exudation of fluid (cerebro spinal) or blood from the nose or ears. Note any unusual odors or mouth discoloration. Check the neck for venous distention, rigidity, and tracheal deviation. The pupils are examined for size and light reaction. Corneal reflexes, ocular motion, conjunctival color, or petechia are checked along with fundiscopic examination. The character of respirations are evaluated, noting any inequality of chest expansion or irregularity of rate. The chest is percussed and auscultated for any evidence of dullness, absence of breath sounds, wheezing, and inspiratory or expiratory rales. The possibility of pleural fluid, blood, or air must be recognized. Percuss the chest for any evidence of cardiac enlargement. Auscultate the heart for rhythm, murmers, or deficits. At the same time, check femoral pulse for evidence of satisfactory perfusion. The abdominal examination must include search for abdominal breathing, distention, organ enlargement, masses, rigidity, bladder distention, and bowel sounds. A rectal examination for blood should be included. Inspect the back for vertebral alignment, injury, or decubite. The extremities must be evaluated from the standpoint of movement, flaccidity, deformity, edema, pulsations, reflexes, and response to stimuli. Neurologic examination including the cranial nerves is mandatory.

LABORATORY STUDIES

The initial blood studies should include sugar, CBC and differential, hematocrit, electrolites, BUN, and blood gases. As mentioned before, it is wise to draw enough blood initially for special studies that might be indicated as more of the clinical diagnosis becomes known. Typing and cross-matching must be considered. Urine should be obtained for analysis, and it is at this time that the patient is usually catheterized. Check urine for blood, sugar, and acetone. Store the specimen for drug level unless such toxins have been ruled out. The use of a gastric tube for gross and chemical analysis as well as lavage and a preventive measure of aspiration is frequently a productive procedure. A lumbar puncture unless contraindicated, such as in the case of a suspected posterior fossa lesion, and the analysis of cerebro spinal fluid and culture can be most useful, particularly in the febrile patient. X-rays are ordered as indicated but not without some clinical lead. Special studies as cerebral angiograms and echograms are performed when the patient is initially stabilized and a working diagnosis such as a central nervous system lesion is suspected.

It is thus seen that an orderly attempt is made to profit by each bit of information as it becomes available and to pursue the investigation along the lines suggested by the findings.

POISONING

Acute poisoning is one of the problems in any emergency department. It must be remembered that those who bring in the victims are likely to have overlooked the need for identifying the poison. They expect the doctors to know what to do. A planned procedure for identifying the poison should be in the procedure manual. This may include a telephone call back to the home or wherever the patient came from or even a quick visit there. The department should have on hand the antidotes for common poisons and an easily interpreted file or card index of antidotes. Unless the department functions as a Poison Information Center, with extensive information on a wide variety of poisons, it should have telephonic communication with such a center. The number to be called should be clearly identified in a prominent place known to all personnel.

As in the case of the comatose patient, treatment to the extent of getting the poison out of the stomach while the nature of the poison is being determined is often indicated. It must never be forgotten that some medications thought of as harmless may be lethal in large doses. Children have died from swallowing large numbers of children's aspirin tablets.

ACUTE MEDICAL INFECTIONS

The departmental procedure manual should clearly outline precautions to be taken in the case of communicable diseases. The attitude toward spread of such diseases is more rational and less subject to panic than it formerly was, but there are still conditions where the diagnosis or suspected diagnosis call for isolation. As stated in Chapter 20, the manual should also include specific instructions regarding legal procedures for reporting such diseases.

REFERENCE

1. Hurry up—but think. *Emergency Medicine*, Aug. 1971, pp. 51–85.

Chapter 17

THE PSYCHIATRIC PATIENT IN THE EMERGENCY DEPARTMENT

Ralph D. Worthylake and C.H. Hardin Branch

An appraisal of the emergency department and its functions from a psychiatric point of view can be approached in at least two ways. The first is the strictly, narrowly psychiatric consideration; the second is with a wider, more inclusive perspective which takes into account some of the sociological, humanitarian, and even philosophical implications of the emergency department and its impact on all individuals who come in contact with it, whether hospital personnel, patient, or friends and relatives of patients. One of the greatest insights in modern psychiatry is the discovery of the importance of the crisis situation and its resolution, and the emergency department is the place par excellence where the crisis-stricken individual comes into first contact with the healing professions. We shall discuss first the physical aspects of the emergency department, both desirable and undesirable, which are pertinent to the psychologically helpful management of the patient; second, a few specific points in the management of psychotic, toxic, depressed, or agitated patients; third, the potential of the emergency department in the training and education of people who take in-hospital training in the medical and paramedical professions; and last, some of the humanitarian factors in the running of an emergency department.

DESIGN

In comparison with some of the other disciplines in medicine, psychiatry makes few hard and fast requirements regard-

275

ing the physical arrangements of the emergency area. To the psychiatrist, the attitudes and behavior of the emergency department personnel in receiving and caring for the psychiatric patient are much more important than the physical setup; however, the design of the emergency department can in many ways influence the psychiatric patient, favorably or unfavorably, and can facilitate or complicate the tasks of the emergency department workers.

In any emergency department, the press of work sometimes requires that patients be placed in a common waiting room until space in treatment or interview rooms becomes available. No matter how heavy the rush, every person applying at the emergency department must be interviewed by intake personnel immediately upon arrival so that the nature of the complaint can be determined. At the very moment of accepting the patient's application, the hospital accepts a legal as well as a moral responsibility for the patient, and therefore the waiting room must be arranged so that those in it can be unobtrusively observed from an adjacent desk or office. People showing evidence of distress or behavior disturbing to others can thus be reported immediately to the head nurse or doctor in charge. To have one of the emergency department workers in sight also helps relieve the waiting patients of any feeling they might have of being neglected or forgotten, and gives them a person readily available to answer questions or to reassure them. If space is available, it might be desirous to have several small waiting rooms instead of one large one, to afford greater privacy for patients and their accompanying family members.

The emergency area should be designed so that ambulance patients need not be brought through the general admission area but can be admitted through a separate entrance and taken immediately to treatment rooms near that entrance. This protects both the dignity of such seriously ill or injured people and the sensibilities of those in the waiting room. Similar admission of seriously disturbed psychotic patients can usually be arranged, since such admissions are almost always preceded by a telephoned announcement of their arrival.

Examination Area

The treatment or examination area should be so arranged that the emotionally disturbed patient can be interviewed and examined in a relatively soundproof room where he can feel free to talk without fearing that he is overheard. Providing ample space in such a room for the presence of one or more family members is desirable, for while an occasional psychiatric patient may prefer to be apart from his family, more are comforted and supported by the presence of familiar people in what is often to them a strange and threatening situation. Such rooms would also be useful for others, such as children and elderly people, to whom the presence of a familiar face is reassuring.

The areas to be encountered by psychiatric patients should be free of any unfamiliar or potentially disturbing equipment, such as sterilizers and x-ray machines, which might lend themselves to delusional ideation or simply cause increased anxiety. Signs should be simple and unambiguous in their wording, and everything should contribute to the feeling of structure and stability. It has been noted, for example, that signs hanging by nearly invisible wires have disturbed psychotic patients, whose contact with reality is already tenuous.

In emergency departments in which patients are placed in adjoining beds or cubicles separated only by curtains or screens, particular attention must be given to acoustical engineering to minimize the arousal of anxiety in some patients by overhearing sounds of distress from others. The facilitation of nursing care through an open arrangement makes it attractive, but the potential for emotional disturbance in the patients must not thereby be minimized. We must turn to the architects and acoustical engineers for resolution of this problem.

Observation Room

It seems highly desirable that the emergency department have some facility, perhaps a small ward, where patients may be kept for observation over a period of as long as eight hours or so, without formal admission to the main wards of the hospital. Frequently (we are thinking of cases of drug ingestion, either accidental or in a suicide gesture where the psychiatrist does not feel that inpatient treatment is indicated), the responsible physician finds himself forced, either by arbitrary rules governing the permitted length of stay in the emergency department or by lack of facilities for observation, into admitting to the main wards of the hospital a patient who realistically needs only observation for a few hours and in whom there is small likelihood of serious developments. Provision for such extended observation would seem to be a natural function of the emergency department; it would enable the physician to make more informed disposition of the problem patient, and would in many cases result in less expense to the patient.

Isolation Room

In hospitals with facilities for psychiatric inpatients, an isolation room in the emergency area is probably not necessary; a person so disturbed as to require isolation almost certainly needs to be admitted to the hospital and can go directly to the psychiatric ward. Hospitals without satisfactory arrangements for disturbed patients may find it advisable to have a room which can be locked for patients who cannot be managed by persuasion and medication. It must be borne in mind, however, that a person who finds himself locked in a room will invariably feel himself rejected and punished and, in proportion as his anger increases and his sense of responsibility for his own actions is diminished, will tend to act upon such feelings. Two general trends of action must be considered and handled: hostility, with aggression toward the physical environment; and aggression toward the self, either from despair or with the intent of creating embarrassment and difficulty for the attending personnel.

To reduce the emotional shock and the implication of rejection and punishment, such a room should be well lighted, with some use of color to make it as attractive as possible, and the use of bars or heavy screens must be strictly avoided. These last features, with their connotation of dangerous criminals and caged beasts only further the dehumanization of an individual who already feels estranged from other people, and frequently such trappings act as goads and challenges to destructive behavior.

To minimize the opportunity for acting out aggressive feelings, the room must be designed so that potentially dangerous features are eliminated insofar as possible. Light fixtures should be recessed into the ceiling and covered with "unbreakable" plastic. The necessary observation window can be made of the same material. Such windows must be kept small; large sheets of such material can be broken and are not suitable for full-size windows. Glass bricks make a not unattractive outside window, but the type of glass brick should be carefully selected; some do transmit distorted or multiple, small images of people or objects on the other side, and these can be quite disturbing to an agitated patient. No projections should be present which might lend themselves to an attempted hanging. Drapery rods, if present at all, should be designed to support little more than the weight of the drapes. Radiators should be housed in wooden guards with sloping tops so that one cannot stand on them, and all sharp projecting corners are to be avoided. The bed should be spot-welded together so that it cannot be disassembled, and the door must be wide enough so that if a strong, violent person uses the entire bed as a weapon, it can be easily removed. Bathroom facilities should be near the isolation room but not opening directly into it, and the hot water taps in such a facility should contain a thermostatic control which regulates the heat of the water delivered to keep it below scalding temperatures.

It seems to us that the disadvantages of equipping the locked room with a two-way communication system far outweigh any possible advantages. Listening is no substitute for the necessary frequent visual observation, and the patient has often had more than enough experience with disembodied voices already. The arrangement, unfortunately, also caters to the callous individual of little empathy and less taste who inclines toward the "this is God" type of sadism.

A patient, upon being put into a locked room, must be

relieved of any personal articles that might be used in a violent manner; this can be done most expeditiously and least punitively by exchanging his street clothing and contents for a hospital gown or pajamas.

It should be mentioned that anyone ordering a person locked in an isolation room or carrying out such an order should be familiar and compliant with the laws of the state concerning commitment procedures and involuntary detention of persons, and should be prepared to justify the action in court, if necessary. There is no substitute for accurate recording in such cases.

PROFESSIONAL ATTITUDE

We have said earlier that the attitude and behavior of the emergency department personnel are, in our opinion, of much greater importance in the care of psychiatric patients than the physical arrangement of the area. The doctor or nurse working with the psychiatric patient must, to be effectively helpful, be able to convey an understanding of the patient's distress, a willingness to be of as much help as is realistically possible, and the assurance that the nature of the problem does not diminish the patient's individual worth and dignity as a person. These attitudes can make it possible for the patient to accept his problem and encourage his realistic handling of it. These attitudes, however, cannot convincingly be imparted if they are not sincerely felt.

Unfortunately, some professional people share in the archaic attitudes of the lay public toward the emotionally disturbed person and lack both the sophistication and the empathy to handle adequately these suffering people. The responsible supervisor must be as quick to detect and correct these episodes of faulty management as he would be if they occurred with medical or surgical patients.

Doubts concerning one's own sanity are very common among people in emotional turmoil, and among the less-sophisticated members of the population the belief is common that doctors are eager to detect signs of derangement in order to commit the victim to a mental institution; this combination of factors, along with the social stigmata of psychiatric illness, are powerful deterrents to seeking help. If, when he does arrive at the emergency department, the emotionally ill person is treated by the personnel as a "crock" who is taking up their valuable time and is probably hopeless anyway, to be brushed off with a placebo or its equivalent, he may retreat to his own methods of problem solving, which may include desertion of his family, abuse of his spouse and children, alcoholism, or suicide. Perhaps only in the field of infectious disease are the adverse effects of illness so regularly harmful to persons other than the designated patient.

Psychotic patients in the emergency department do demand certain kinds of treatment, which should be emphasized. The highly suspicious, paranoid patient who feels that he has been brought to the emergency department by whatever malign forces are surrounding him, can best be handled by a matter-of-fact statement of the situation as it exists, including the legal side of the picture. Some reassurance can be provided if he is offered an immediate opportunity to get in touch with his lawyer, clergyman, or such members of the family as are not perceived as part of the "plot" against him. The physician and the rest of the personnel must be very sure that they do not accept his delusional statements as true, and at the same time it is useless to try to "talk him out of it." It is worse than useless and even cruel to buy time by pretending to agree with his psychotic thinking. As an example, if the patient states that he is hearing voices and asks the physician if he doesn't hear them, the proper response is not, "Yes, I hear them, too," in an attempt to placate the patient, but rather, "No, I do not hear them myself, but apparently something is disturbing you."

Restraints vs Medication

About the use of restraints—in psychiatric treatment facilities they are very rarely used. It is probably desirable to have available a set of padded, leather wrist and ankle restraints, but if they are used more frequently than once in a year or two in the average emergency department, it is presumptive evidence that the emergency department care of psychiatric patients needs careful reevaluation. The effects of good interpersonal relationship were described in 1842 by Charles Dickens following a visit to the Boston Lunatic Hospital. He stated: "Moral influence alone restrains the more violent among them, but the effect of that influence is one hundred times more efficacious than all the strait waistcoats, fetters and handcuffs that ignorance, prejudice and cruelty have manufactured since the creation of the world." In passing, it should be noted that police handcuffs, used on struggling, agitated individuals, have resulted in severe nerve damage. The judicious use of medication, particularly the phenothiazine derivatives, has largely done away with the need for restraints and, to a lesser degree, for seclusion. The emergency department physician should be well informed in the use of such medications or avail himself of immediate consultation concerning them rather than subject the patient to restraints unnecessarily.

As a point of diagnostic distinction for those who may have had limited contact with severely disturbed patients, the presence of obvious confusion, disorientation, and misidentification of other people is *not* characteristic of functional illness, and should alert the physician to seek carefully for an organic or metabolic etiological agent.

One of the commonest types of psychiatric patient to come to the emergency department is the person who has attempted suicide or made a suicide gesture, or the individual who is brought in by concerned relatives or friends because of the fear of suicide. Evaluating the risk in such persons is one of the heaviest responsibilities in psychiatry, and if psychiatric consultation is available it should always be obtained in such cases before final disposition is made. Pending such evaluation, the emergency department doctor will have to form some opinion as to the severity of the risk; if he feels it is grave, the greatest protection that can be given is not to place the patient in isolation, but to provide him with a *constant* attendant. A person determined to destroy himself can be remarkably ingenious, and the practice of "checking" the patient every ten to fifteen minutes, while common, does not provide maximum protection. Many patients have killed or seriously injured themselves in the interim between "checks."

It should be noted that the attendant in this situation need not necessarily be a registered nurse or even a licensed practical nurse. This could well be the kind of responsibility which could be entrusted to a volunteer or to paid medical, social work, or psychology students or others who might find it a rewarding experience as well as a lucrative one. The important thing is to have someone there who can forestall the suicide attempts of a patient and can call for help if this should be needed. A buzzer or other unobtrusive call system should be in operation for getting help so that the attendant need not leave the patient.

Especially careful attention should be paid to those individuals who may be on drugs like Antabuse, when the odor of alcohol on the breath and the severe physical prostration may make the hasty physician feel that he is dealing with a case of alcoholic intoxication, whereas actually the situation is far more serious. Any patient receiving Antabuse should carry in his wallet a card stating this fact, warning any physician who sees him that the presence of an alcoholic breath may not indicate in his case the presence of an alcohol intoxication. In these, as in other emergency department situations, adequate volunteer and social work help is essential to the process of identifying the individual and finding the warnings which may be carried on the person or in his wallet.

In all psychiatric cases seen in the emergency department, the patients should be given specific directions as to where definitive help may be obtained. In many areas, due to lack of facilities, this may amount only to the giving of names of one or more psychiatrists in the nearest city, but in no case should a patient with emotional problems be discharged with the impression that there is nothing that can be done for him. The emergency department physician may at times feel certain that the patient will not follow through with the recommendation, and he may well be right; that is the patient's privilege, but he should have the best available advice nonetheless.

Since friends or members of the patient's family often accompany him to the emergency department, some thought should be given to their needs. It should be possible in any emergency department for such relatives or friends to obtain food, either from the hospital cafeteria or from vending machines in the emergency department area or adjacent to it. Similarly, provision should be made for a telephone accessible to patients and relatives. Adequate coverage by social workers should be provided around the clock in the emergency departments of larger hospitals; often the fact that not very much occurs at night seems to justify minimal social work coverage because it is not economically practical. Anyone, however, who has seen small children forlornly waiting in the room, bewildered, hungry, thirsty, afraid, or ashamed to ask for help in getting to the toilet, etc., must feel that economic considerations are much less important than providing for the creature comforts of these unfortunate and frightened individuals. At the very least, social workers in the hospital can be placed on an emergency call system just like other professional personnel. A well-trained social worker can arrange foster home care, obtain transportation home, and notify helpful relatives, but these responsibilities cannot be added to the burdens of the emergency department personnel whose chief responsibility it is to administer to the medical, surgical, or psychiatric needs of the outpatient. This whole area has a definite significance when it comes to the patient himself, and no one who has been a patient in an emergency department can forget the worry he has about whether the creature comforts of his relatives are being taken care of.

EDUCATION

The emergency department also has, we feel, a much greater potential role in the educational program of the hospital than is usually assigned to it. It has long been the excellent practice to give interns and some resident house officers the experience of serving a part of their training time there, but is there not considerable value to be derived from the experience for other disciplines that give part of their training in the hospital, such as the psychology students, social work trainees, and student nurses? One nurse of our acquaintance said that she had had six weeks of her training in the diet kitchen, but only two weeks in the emergency department, which she felt indicated a priority rating of some kind. This is not to argue that persons in all the above-named disciplines need to acquire specific emergency department skills, but too often their training programs as usually constituted provide scant or no opportunity for getting a good perspective of the problems that face the physician on his first contact with the patient; the task, for example, of deciding whether the disturbed, confused patient is suffering from a metabolic upset such as insulin reaction, from a toxic reaction to chemicals or drugs, or from a functional condition. Observing at first hand the scope of the physician's role should add greatly to the trainee's perspective of medicine in general and psychiatry in particular, and can help to further a feeling of community of purpose in service to the patient.

It is not inconceivable that such individuals might not only be of immediate help in the emergency department but might be able to contribute something to the physician's understanding of the behavior of people in crises and the difference in response to crisis of people of different classes and conditions, which would be of permanent value to him in his profession.

In hospitals associated with medical schools, the emergency department should be considered a vital part of the education of the medical students. From the psychiatric point of view, it offers students not only a first contact with psychiatric patients but also an opportunity to observe in an emergency situation those psychic elements which complicate or confuse medical and surgical illnesses. The student should learn to be familiar with the histrionic and overdramatic recital of symptoms which is characteristic of the patient with a conversion reaction, the kinds of physical findings which are associated with hysterical episodes, and the overreaction to an injury or to a symptom which may suggest that the patient has had actual or vicarious experience with this same symptom previously and is overreacting to it because of a functional overlay rather than because of the symptom itself. In this connection it is essential to note that many people, in spite of column after column of medical information in the daily press, are still incredibly naive about their own anatomy and physiology and may be realistically reacting to an injury or illness as they understand the mechanisms inside their bodies. The physician must, wherever possible, reassure the individual as to the actual difficulties; a certain amount of help should be given to the family members who may be present and who will, in their turn, help reassure the patient. This is particularly applicable in the case of young children where the terror of a mother may be transmitted to the child, with resultant actual damage to the latter. Reassurance of the mother by the physician may result in an appropriate calming effect on the child.

HUMANITARIAN ASPECT

The emergency department is an excellent classroom for what may be called the humanitarian and even the romantic aspects of medicine. There has been a great deal of concern recently about the loss of the image of the physician, and to some extent the creation of marvellous technical equipment has depreciated the role of the physician as a human being. It is in the emergency department that this role should be most dramatically underlined, and it is for this reason that we feel very strongly that all individuals who receive any part of their training in a hospital should see in pure culture the stricken patient, the frightened members of the family, and the other social forces, including police officers and ambulance personnel, which impinge upon the situation. It is here that these personnel should learn how a realistic, matter-of-fact, kindly, reassuring point of view cannot only be of tremendous benefit for the psychologic needs of the patient, but may actually be lifesaving.

It is true that some emergency departments are misused. The fact that a private physician can often not keep an appointment for several weeks may make the patient "drop by" the emergency department in order to get medication, the refill of a prescription, or something of that sort. In fact, some physicians are inclined to use the emergency department for just this purpose. Perhaps it would help curtail this practice if the emergency departments in most hospitals had printed forms advising the patient and his physician that this is a misuse of the emergency department, that the patient had a right to expect certain service from his personal physician, and that it is both unfair and unwise to use the emergency department for purposes for which it was not intended.

In the small-town hospital, the emergency department has a difficult role to play. It is often quite impossible to staff it on a round-the-clock basis, and in many instances the only staff which can be provided will be a nurse who will come from another part of the hospital when someone pushes a buzzer. She, in turn, is responsible for locating a physician who will come to the hospital. It might be possible in such a small town to obtain around-the-clock service by use of volunteers from the community. Certainly, during the war it was possible to find a great number of people who could give up some of their time on a rotation basis to man ambulances or emergency stations of one kind or another, and local volunteer organizations might, on a rotation basis, assume the responsibility of actually staying in the emergency department on this sort of schedule. A cool-headed person with even a minimum of first-aid training could certainly keep the situation from getting worse until the nurse could be summoned, and it would have the advantage of involving the community actively in the emergency department program.

It may be "old hat" to think nostalgically of the days when emergency department activities were the most dramatic part of the hospital, but it does appear to be true that the present day of bowing to the very real domestic responsibilities of the medical students and thus cutting down their ability to "drop by the emergency department" takes away something from the practice of medicine as they visualized it when they entered school. It has been repeatedly pointed out that many medical students have reported that the humanitarian interest they had in medicine when they came into the medical school had been lost and they had become less concerned with people as individuals as they progressed through the medical curriculum. The emergency department could very well be an excellent place for them to learn the many ways in which people can be heroic in the face of adversity, can tolerate tragedies with equanimity, and really rise to great spiritual heights. Also, in this same setting, the student physician can learn that he alone may represent the difference between terror and reassurance and, in the patient's mind, the difference between life and death. Whether or not this is literally true, it is for many students the reason for which they came into medicine, and it would be unfortunate if this part of medical practice were limited to the television screen and the stage. There is sufficient drama in any emergency department to satisfy all of the perfectly justifiable needs of the young physician for reassurance that he is in a profession which has a certain aura of greatness about it. It is here that he can learn that in spite of the technological advances of medicine and surgery, in many patients' minds it is still the physician as a human being who stands between him and the terrors of the dark.

Chapter 18

THE EMERGENCY DEPARTMENT
AS AN EDUCATIONAL CENTER

Difficulties are frequently encountered in gaining staff support for regular trauma conferences in community hospitals. It is not suggested that the Joint Commission on Accreditation of Hospitals add this to its requirements of staff meetings, but such conferences, well planned and regularly held, have more effect on reduction of mortality and morbidity than some of the required exercises.

The trend toward specialism tends to divide doctors into strictly segregated groups that neither know much nor care much about medical problems outside their named specialties. The term "specialist," as applied to the medical profession, has been defined in various ways. The author has defined it as "a doctor from another town." This definition is based partially on the attitude of some patients. It is also said that a specialist is a doctor who claims to know nothing about anything outside his own specialty. This may be a successful way for the young specialist to set himself apart, but it is a negative approach and does not stamp him as a very good doctor.*

It will be a long time until state boards of medical examiners

---

* This would be a good place for me to make a confession. In the course of my oral American Board of Surgery examination, the subject of peptic ulcer came up. I seemed to do all right in stating my criteria for advocating surgical treatment. One of the examiners then asked me how I would manage a patient with ulcer who did not qualify for surgery. Knowing that both of the examiners were from teaching hospitals where there were "all sorts and conditions of famous physicians" (with thanks to A.A. Milne), I replied without hesitation, "Oh, I would refer him to a gastroenterologist." This seemed to satisfy the two professors and they switched the questioning to other subjects. What I didn't tell them was that I was the gastroenterologist to whom I would refer the patient, because there were no gastroenterologists on the hospital staff or in my community. It is the responsibility of the surgeon to try to keep the patient out of the operating room if he can safely and rationally do so, and there is some question whether the surgeon who does not understand the medical management of peptic ulcer should do gastric surgery.

cease licensing medical graduates to practice medicine and surgery. Until they do, a lot of people will continue to look to the average M.D. for help in emergencies. A little knowledge of what to do will not tarnish the reputation of any specialist. Certainly, any physician who poses as a family doctor or a surgeon should be able to provide immediate care in the average emergency. The surgeon should not completely dodge the medical emergency. The early management of such things as coronary occlusion, diabetic coma, insulin shock, ingestion of poisons, to name a few, is standard enough that even a surgeon can start procedures in the right direction prior to obtaining more expert help. By the same token, the internist will not reduce his stature by acquainting himself with such procedures as tracheostomy, application of a Thomas splint, or the giving of intravenous blood or dextran to a severely injured patient.

Discussions of these acute medical and surgical problems should be a regular feature of staff or departmental meetings. To make the internist feel more welcome, the term "emergency conference" might be substituted for "trauma conference." Case reports from actual experience in the emergency department, both medical and surgical, are the framework on which such discussions are built. They are of more value than some things discussed at the standard clinical-pathological conferences. (See reference to death audits in Chapter 8.)

Rapid strides are being made in eliminating some of the scourges affecting human health. This applies, for the most part, to pathological conditions with insidious onset. Little is being done to reduce the incidence of emergencies, and they are increasing and will continue to increase in the foreseeable future. This disturbs many physicians and it should concern them all. This concern should lead them to covet the ability to render help in these emergencies. The satisfaction that accrues from rendering such service can only be appreciated by those who have experienced it. Emergencies are not planned and, for this reason, come as a shock to the victims. Their sense of gratitude for expert care is oftentimes increased for this very reason. "The injured citizen will sing your praises and oftentimes pay your bill."[1]

In a previous chapter it has been clearly stated that emergency room care should not be downgraded but should be provided by physicians skilled in the required techniques. But it is surprising how the expert care of certain emergencies can be taught in the emergency department in a short time. No doubt, the surgical departments of all medical schools teach the proper treatment of lacerations, but it is surprising how such teaching is forgotten and replaced by concerns of lesser importance. Many a young graduate, through his internship and possibly his residency, will center his medical abilities on trying to determine whether his hopelessly doomed chronic alcoholic patient has a liver surface that resembles a hobnailed boot or a crepe-soled shoe and feel he is doing his teachers proud. This mental exercise is not likely to do anything for his patient, although it may call attention to the erudition of the young graduate. If he is on a hospital staff where he takes a turn in the emergency department, he might well cease his cerebrations about the liver and drop by the emergency room to watch some of his more experienced and practical colleagues deal with lacerations. If by watching them he relearns that dirty wounds need thorough irrigation and meticulous debridement before suturing, he will know something that will really increase his value to the community. If he happens to come from one of the medical schools which neglect to teach the proper splinting of long-bone fractures, he may learn something in his own emergency department that will be valuable in reducing morbidity and disability from these injuries. He will at least learn not to discourage expert laymen from applying good first aid at the road side, a practice not unknown among doctors not versed in emergency care. The stories that are told of the impotence of some of the products of our great citadels of surgical training, when confronted with victims of traumatic injuries, are discouraging to say the least. They may correct this deficiency by an informal postgraduate course in the emergency department of the hospital where they elect to practice, but only if they have the will to learn.

Several groups of people may profit from practical instruction in the emergency department. These include medical students, interns, residents, members of the attending staff, nurses, and members of ambulance crews.

Cole[2] has pointed out that all medical students should have the opportunity to serve in an emergency room. He explains that in conjunction with the MEND (Medical Education for National Defense) program, freshmen medical students at the University of Illinois College of Medicine have a series of twelve lectures on emergency care, mostly at the first aid level. They are also encouraged to spend time in the emergency department, particularly at night. When they become seniors, they are assigned to the emergency department in two's to serve from 6:00 P.M. until midnight or later, for four to six sessions but not on successive nights. They are again encouraged to visit the emergency department on other evenings when their schedule allows.

Interns may profit by regularly assigned periods of duty in the emergency department. While this may be considered a period of instruction through practical experience, the intern should not be given a free reign. If he is conscientious, he will want advice and help from someone more experienced. If he is not, he will need it all the more. A resident from the appropriate service should be called when the patient has any complaint of much severity. The resident may instruct the intern to carry on with the treatment, but only in line with the resident's judgment.

Residents should be assigned to emergency department call for periods of at least several months, but they must also be encouraged to call a member of the attending staff, similarly assigned, if they do not feel fully confident of the diagnosis and management of the emergency. As time goes on, both the intern and the resident will become capable of bearing greater responsibility and will need less supervision. No emergency department, however, should depend on interns alone for professional coverage.

Even though members of the attending staff will have the final responsibility when they are on call, many of them may augment their education in this department. Consultations are educational whether called for by staff regulation or because the doctor feels the need of help. For the hospital staff which is progressive enough to have a plan of continuing medical education, the emergency department offers a splendid medium for instruction in trauma and other emergencies. It also offers the young surgeon with sufficient formal training to have surgical privileges a place to exploit his talents. While he is passing through the period of establishment in the community, he can make many contacts among both the profession and laymen.

A large majority of emergency departments are in hospitals having neither medical students, interns, nor residents to profit by the educational environment, but this should not negate the learning opportunity. If the staff has accepted the responsibility to improve this service, learning should be part of the program. Well-kept emergency records, supplemented by in-patient records when patients are admitted, offer valuable material for studying the quality of care and for assessing end results in the more severe cases. These may form the basis for stimulating and interesting emergency conferences. The quality of these is not dependent on size. In fact, as hospitals grow and staffs become larger, the valuable effects of small informal conferences are sometimes lost. Long before some of the present day meetings became mandatory, the author used to attend regularly the monthly staff meetings in a hospital of 125 beds. About 30 to 45 minutes of the meeting time was devoted to a review of the x-rays of the fractures of the previous month. There was free discussion, constructive criticism, and a true spirit of learning. These have long since been replaced by many time-consuming meetings that may be of less value.

The learning opportunities in the emergency department are not limited to medical students and doctors. Nurses, to fill the role required in this department, cannot be assigned haphazardly, and they must be trained. With the current trend in nursing education away from practical patient care, few nurses on graduation are ready for assignment to the operating room or an emergency department. Owens[3] states that in Colorado he found that some ambulance attendants complained that, on occasion, the nurses knew less than they, the attendants, did when they arrived at the hospital with injured patients. This situation may be corrected by training after graduation. If the hospital has a training school and a directress of nurses aware of operating room and emergency room needs, she may rotate student nurses through these places and, in doing so, find out which nurses have a bent for this type of work. Some are not fitted for it. To others, it has great appeal.

Whether student or graduate, a nurse should work in this department under supervision of a senior before she is given full responsibility. This is particularly true before she is given a night-shift assignment. She can learn sterile techniques, the preparation for reparative surgery, the location of equipment and supplies, and lifesaving procedures to augment what may have been done before the patient's arrival at the hospital. She must learn more than this, however. As Owens[4] has pointed out, "Her decisions must be rapid; she must be able to screen patients and possess knowledge not only of how to assist in all types of emergency care, but also how to deal with human relations under stress."

It is the responsibility of the doctor in the emergency department to supervise the nurse and aid in her instruction. This should be done with patience and understanding. Loud and unreasonable complaints about unsatisfactory service will gain little. If a nurse fails to respond to instruction and repeatedly renders substandard assistance, her shortcomings should be reported to her superiors and, if necessary, her transfer suggested. The type of nurse who should be assigned here is described in the chapter on staffing. If she has the basic interest and motivation she will become proficient under instruction. She may graduate from the emergency department to the operating room, for the qualities that make for success in these two departments are similar.

Finally, the emergency department is a splendid area in which to check the proficiency of ambulance attendants and to augment their education. The condition in which patients arrive at the emergency department entrance is usually a good index of the first-aid abilities of those who have brought them, but not always. Unfortunately, there are doctors who, through ignorance, interfere with adequate splinting and other proper first-aid measures. They take the attitude of the unsophisticated layman, that the most urgent need is to "rush the patient to the hospital." This reflects on either the doctor's basic training or his ability to use what he was taught. Before an ambulance crew is taken to task for not properly preparing a patient for transportation, it should be determined whether their efforts have been interfered with.

Most ambulance attendants want to do a good job, although some seem disinterested. When a patient with a long-bone fracture is brought in without splinting, there is an excellent opportunity to demonstrate splint application to the ambulance attendants. It should be done promptly, before the patient is subject to transfer, and the reasons for splinting should be explained. Of course, this should not be done in such a way as to give the conscious patient or his family or friends the idea that he has been mishandled.

Ambulance attendants should be made welcome in the emergency department and treated courteously. The great majority will respond to such treatment, will profit by instruction, and will improve the quality of their patient handling.

Seldom should a day go by when someone doesn't learn something worthwhile in a well-run emergency department.

By no means of minor importance is the place that the emergency department itself may play in the education of the public as to its proper use. Most people are reasonable and will respond to the "friendly persuasion" mentioned under methods of education in English hospitals in Chapter 1.

REFERENCES

1. Spencer, J.H.: Please call a doctor. *Bull Am Coll Surgeons,* 1954.
2. Cole, W.H., and Schneewind, J.H.: Teaching of trauma at a university hospital. *Bull Am Coll Surgeons, 40:*204–206, 1955.
3. Owens, J.C.: Personal communication.
4. Owens, J.C.: *Survey of Emergency Departments in Colorado.* A study under a Public Health Service grant, University of Colorado Medical Center, 1965.

Chapter 19

EVALUATION—EMERGENCY
DEPARTMENT SURVEYS

At the 1954 Clinical Congress of the American College of Surgeons, the problem of reducing the annual 12,000 deaths and 1,250,000 injuries from automobile accidents in this country was a major topic of interest. In the annual Oration on Trauma, Dr. Robert H. Kennedy[1] stated, "There is little doubt in my mind that the weakest link in the chain of hospital care in most hospitals in this country, is the emergency room attention to the injured." He asked some pointed questions: "In the emergency room in your hospital, who examines the injured person first? May it be the most junior intern, who has never seen a traumatic case before, or an indifferently trained foreign physician with language difficulty? Have you prepared and posted a directive which will give the junior men an idea of what instances require the immediate notification of a surgical resident?"

"In the middle of the night will this be a resident who has been instructed how to recognize the signs of intra-abdominal injury, for instance, and to call a member of the attending staff now and not wait until tomorrow morning?" He asked other thought-provoking questions, the last one being, "Do you know from personal inspection what goes on in your emergency room in the middle of the night, or do you stay away due to a subconscious fear of what you might see?"

Kennedy concluded with some recommendations, including that of a thorough overhauling of the present concept of the importance of the emergency room in hospital care. In spite of this forthright statement and the challenge issued in 1954, it is difficult to find any evidence of any follow-up action until 1957. Although Kennedy had not referred to it, considerable attention was given during those three years to the growing number of

296

patients coming to emergency departments for all kinds of medical attention. Speeches were made and papers were published with suggestions on how to prepare for this surging tide of general medical problems. There was a singular lack of any effort to correct the deficiencies so eloquently pointed out by Kennedy.

However, in 1957, a small group of New Jersey surgeons interested in better care of the injured did something about it. They accepted the challenge issued in 1954. Led by Dr. S.T. Snedecor, of Hackensack, then Chairman of the New Jersey Committee on Trauma of the American College of Surgeons, they devised a plan of surveying emergency departments in New Jersey hospitals.* This was not a study to write a report on New Jersey hospitals or to classify them as bad, fair, or good. It was a plan of sharing interests through surveys by teams from other hospitals, teams which were in a position to see things objectively. At first, a team of two surgeons and one administrator from three different hospitals visited the emergency department of a fourth hospital and reviewed its activities from all angles. This included location, construction, equipment, professional staffing, nursing service, and anything else that came to mind. As a guide, a questionnaire was prepared and sent in advance to the administrator of the host hospital so that information wanted by the survey team would be available. These surveys were a joint project of the American College of Surgeons' New Jersey Committee on Trauma and the New Jersey Hospital Association. It was made clear that the surveys were not related to any program of accreditation and that information on no hospital would be publicized in connection with the name of the hospital. The report of the survey team was sent back to the administrator of the hospital surveyed, with constructive suggestions for improving the emergency department service. Later, a nurse was added to survey teams, as it was realized that she could gather information and offer suggestions that others might overlook.

Before long, a picture of the emergency department service

* The first survey team was made up of two past chairmen of the New Jersey Committee on Trauma, Doctor Herbert A. Schulte of Newark, Doctor James H. Spencer of Newton (the author), and Doctor Snedecor. Later an administrator was added to the teams.

in New Jersey hospitals began to take shape and confirmed the need for such a study, but the initial purpose of the surveys was not forgotten. Written and verbal reports from some of these hospitals indicate the tremendous value of these surveys. One of the hospitals surveyed in the early stages of the program was a busy one of 110 beds. It had an emergency department consisting of one 12′ × 14′ room. An examining table discarded from elsewhere in the hospital was the only stretcher on which to treat patients. Equipment and supplies were limited and poorly stored. There was no nurse in the emergency department unless one was called from upstairs, and when she was called there was no assurance that she was capable of dealing with emergency situations. The weakest link in the whole program, however, was poor staffing. To be sure, there was a rotating roster of the active staff physicians, with one doctor on first call and another on second for periods of a month at a time, but no attempt had been made to assure that one of these was a surgeon.

There had been a shake-up in staff administration over a year before, breaking a long period of disinterest in progressive staff organization and patient care. After the changes in staff administration, a much needed change was brought about in hospital administration. For the first time, it became possible to introduce progressive and fresh ideas. The idea of an emergency department survey appealed to the new administrator, although he had only been at the helm four months. It was requested, and a survey team was sent by the New Jersey Trauma Committee. The results were revolutionary. The changes brought about following the report from the survey team were not all new ideas. Some of them had been suggested before, but it took a report from disinterested outsiders to get action. The changes included the following:

Moving into new quarters over twice the size of the small room.

Installation of sliding curtains giving privacy to three patients at a time.

Purchase of three new stretchers designed for emergency department use.

Construction of carefully planned cabinets of adequate capacity to hold all supplies (with only the narcotics cabinet kept locked!).

Purchase of anesthesia and resuscitation equipment for use only in the emergency department.

Installation of adequate lighting.

Purchase of much new equipment, such as surgical instruments, and the discarding of substandard equipment.

Assembly of equipment on special trays for such procedures as tracheostomy, thoractomy, spinal puncture, etc., and the clear marking of these before storage in the cabinets.

Establishment of a continuous inventory file of emergency department supplies.

Establishment of a poison control facility, with antidote information and telephone contact with a state poison control center.

Printing of new emergency department record forms with adequate, color-coded copies for all needs.

The establishment of full-time, around-the-clock nursing service by nurses selected for and interested in this type of work.

A complete change in the type of staffing roster with duty periods reduced to two weeks, and to one week in the three summer months; the new roster always had a member of the surgical staff on either first or second call.

It could not be said that every survey had as salutary an effect as this one, but some places did not need as much done. The task was made much easier as a result of changes in hospital administration and in the nursing office, that had taken plcae after the shake-up in staff administration.

Let the Director of Surgery in another New Jersey hospital tell what happened after the survey of his emergency department. He wrote, "I think that your investigation of the Emergency Room at ——— Hospital was extremely fruitful. I think the manner in which it was conducted was most helpful in that it consisted of an on-the-spot investigation by people whose problems in their own hospitals were similar to our own, so the investigation was a sympathetic one. First, it put the personnel through their paces in response to the specific questions addressed to the committee, and second, it caused the committee from the hospital to observe the trial run at a time when all the advantages and disadvantages were seen simultaneously. The net effect of the entire thing was really to provide stimulus to the local group to reexamine the situation in the Emergency Room. . . . it was made the discussion of an Executive Committee meeting and this committee in turn appointed a Trauma Committee which reviewed all the procedures in the Emergency Room and set up a procedure book which is now in the hands of each of the house staff."

He continues by outlining further results at the medical staff level. A review of deaths from trauma in that hospital has been started to cover a period of five years. Unrecognized causes of death as shown at autopsy are particularly being looked for in this review. A meeting of the general surgical department has been devoted to a "review of the priorities of multiple injuries." The director of surgery adds, ". . . it may be that we may set up the system of compulsory consultation or perhaps we can demonstrate the situation convincingly enough so that it will be adopted on a voluntary basis."

It is interesting to note that the first of these two hospitals is a small one in a rural county seat; the second has 450 beds, is in one of New Jersey's largest cities, and has a complete intern and residency training program.

The success of this survey program of the New Jersey Committee on Trauma attracted the interest of the parent group, the Committee on Trauma of the American College of Surgeons.* It set out to do something about emergency departments. The initial approach was somewhat different from that of the New Jersey committee. Rather than a program of national surveys to help the individual hospital, the focus was directed on regional sampling of the state of emergency rooms across the country.

A Field Program of the Committee on Trauma was instituted, under a grant from the John A. Hartford Foundation in 1960. A

* The author was invited to present the program to the Committee.

study of the emergency room problem in North America was selected as its major project.

At the same time that the New Jersey Committee was activating its program, the American Hospital Association was reactivating its Committee on Hospital Outpatient Services. This committee chose the emergency department as the facility most urgently needing attention. The American College of Surgeons joined forces with the American Hospital Association in co-sponsoring the regional sampling. This study was carried out by the Cornell University Medical College Trauma Research Group, aided by a United States Public Health Research Grant. Scudder, McCarroll, and Wade[2] published the findings of this study in 1961 along with some pertinent recommendations. Reference to this study will be found in Chapter 2 under the discussion of location of the department.

Another regional study was carried out by Owens[3] in Colorado. He visited 72 general hospitals varying in size from 14 to 475 beds. He reported that 51 of these, or 71 percent, had less than 100 beds. He points out that other reports have been "heavily weighted by observations in larger hospitals." His report is particularly valuable because it is representative of the majority of hospitals in this country. It is worthy of study by anyone wanting to see a picture of the emergency department in the average hospital in the United States. Several references to his findings are made elsewhere in this book.

While this sampling of the state of emergency departments in selected areas across the country was being done, the Committee on Trauma through the Field Program and through the state and provincial committees was attempting to institute individual personal surveys of emergency departments. Lacking the proper liaison with state hospital associations, this program did not spread as widely as might have been hoped. Steps have now been taken by the Subcommittee on Emergency Room Standards of the Committee on Trauma to establish this liaison. A series of group conferences in connection with regional hospital associations has been started.

Hospital administrators are showing an interest, and they are being urged to contact the American College of Surgeons state trauma chairmen to request such surveys. At the same time, the state and provincial trauma chairmen are being urged to work with the hospital associations to accomplish this aim. This program, if it is to have its maximum impact in upgrading emergency department care, must be a joint effort of surgeons and administrators. It is worth mentioning again that the plan has no connection with any accreditation program. It is purely a sharing of mutual efforts to offer every hospital the benefit of objective and constructive criticism. The value of such surveys to the individual hospital has been proven beyond a doubt. Furthermore, they benefit the members of the survey teams who see features that will help their own institutions.

Any group of interested people connected with a hospital could make a survey of its own emergency department, but a survey done by outsiders may prove more objective and effective. It is to be hoped that administrators of hospitals requesting such surveys will be willing to serve on teams going to other institutions.

Hospitals interested in availing themselves of this service should communicate with the chairman of the American College of Surgeons Committee on Trauma in the state or province. If any difficulty is experienced in getting his name through any Fellow of the College, this information is available from the Secretary to the Committee on Trauma, American College of Surgeons, 55 East Erie Street, Chicago, Illinois, 60611.

The checklist used by the New Jersey committee is reproduced here to show the thoroughness with which these surveys have been done.

HOSPITAL EMERGENCY ROOM SURVEY
QUESTION CHECK LIST

I. VOLUME of WORK
  Total of Patients:_____
  1. Traumatic_____
  2. Surgical_____
  3. Medical_____
  4. Miscellaneous_____
II. ORGANIZATION of TRAUMA SERVICE
  1. Which service has responsibility for Emergency Room?

2. Team Organization.
   a. How does it function?
   b. When are Attendings called?
   c. Which service has charge of Multiple Injuries?
   d. Who is captain of team?
   e. Who calls consultations of different services?
3. Standard Operating Procedures.
   Each service; for example, eye, foreign bodies, E.N.T., nose bleeds, general surgery, abdominal trauma?
4. Standards of Practice. Who has responsibility for supervision of doctors using Emergency Room?
   a. General Practitioners.
   b. Compensation Doctors.
   c. Various Specialists.
5. Provisions for Special Types of Cases.
   a. Burns.
   b. Hands.
   c. Shock.
      Availability of blood.
   d. Fractures.
      How are they handled?
      Who may reduce fractures?
      What fractures do interns reduce? Are they supervised?
      Are postoperative X-rays taken on all cases?
      What fractures are admitted?
      Who has supervision of fracture surgery?
      Who approves reductions?

III. PERSONNEL
   A. Attending Staff.
      1. What services are represented?
      2. Qualifications.
      3. Daily attending call list.
      4. Assignment of cases.
      5. Consultation.
   B. Interns-Residents.
      1. Adequate assignment at all hours.
      2. Training—reliability and responsibility.
      3. Teaching—supervision, instruction guides, etc.
   C. Nurses—R.N.'s
      1. Adequate coverage at all hours.
      2. Proper supervision.
      3. Special training.
   D. Practical Nurses—Aides.
   E. Orderlies.
      Training.

F. Volunteers—First Aiders.

G. Extra help—all categories, when needed.

IV. PHYSICAL FACILITIES
1. Reception area.
2. Examination, treatment rooms.
3. Screens in rooms.
4. Minor operating rooms.
5. Fracture, plaster room.
6. Observation or overnight rooms.
7. Waiting rooms for relatives.
8. Storage space.
9. Communication system.
10. Scrubbing facilities.
   a. Doctors.
   b. Patients.
11. Relation to:
   a. X-ray.
   b. Pharmacy.
   c. Laboratory.
   d. Central supply.

V. EQUIPMENT
1. Stretchers (adequate number and type).
2. Wheel chairs.
3. Operating tables.
4. Lighting.
5. Rest beds.
6. Oxygen.
7. Suction.
8. Resuscitation.
9. Defibrillator.
10. Tracheostomy.
11. Gastric lavage set-up.
12. Catheter set-up.
13. Instruments (selection and quality for different types of surgery).
14. Types of sutures.
15. Splints—slings.
16. Bandages—muslin—elastic—adhesive.
17. Linen for drapes, towels.
18. Masks, caps, gowns.
19. Incidental equipment basins, syringes, etc.
20. Burn packages.
21. Intravenous fluids and equipment: Dextran-plasma-glucose, Cut down sets.

  22. Medications.
      a. Stimulants.
      b. Antiseptics.
      c. Biologicals.
      d. Antibiotics.
      e. Sedatives.
      f. Other drugs.

VI. SPECIAL SERVICES
  A. X-ray.
    1. Availability.
    2. Reading of emergency films.
    3. Night and week end coverage.
  B. Laboratory.
    Availability for emergency tests.
  C. Anesthesia.
    1. General availability and quality for fractures, etc.
    2. Local—solutions used, instructions for interns.

VII. PROCESSING of PATIENTS
  A. Reception—Technique.
  B. Information—Registration.
  C. Charts (Are they written before patient leaves emergency room?) Special Emergency Traumatic Charts.
  D. Adequate treatment period in emergency room.
    1. Until shock is relieved.
    2. To O. R. when ready.
    3. Observation.
  E. Admission of Patients.
  F. Routine work-up.
  G. Fracture Patients (proper splinting, handling, discharge instructions).
  H. Discharge of patients.
    1. Clearance by:
      a. Interns.
      b. Attending.
    2. Instructions to patients.
      a. Own doctor.
      b. Staff doctor.
      c. Clinic.
      d. Pamphlet.

VIII. SPECIAL INSTRUCTIONS ON:
  A. D.O.A.
  B. Alcoholics.
  C. Mental Cases.
  D. Suicides.

IX. CHARGES
   A. What are the usual hospital charges?
       Are they adequate and responsible for good service?
   B. Does hospital differentiate clearly between
       hospital service and surgical?
   C. Are Attending Surgeons permitted to charge?
       What cases?
   D. How are compensation cases assigned?

If a questionnaire such as the foregoing were to be used alone, it would not have the effect that it has along with a team survey. The knowledge that a survey team is going to personally visit the department will act as a deterrent against less than frank replies to the questions on the checklist. The Committee on Outpatient Services of the American Hospital Association felt that some of their questionnaire reports were not completely dependable. This lack of dependability corresponds to that seen in some of the surveys that have been made on transportation of the injured. The accuracy of these depends on the objectivity of the person answering the questions. If he happens to be the chief of a fire department who is sincerely interested in improving an ambulance service for which he is responsible, he will admit the shortcomings. If he is simply trying to impress the mayor and the city council, he may not.

The reason that on-the-spot surveys of emergency departments by impartial teams from elsewhere are more effective than mailed questionnaires is that they are done with nothing in mind but helping the hospital surveyed. However, if a medical staff or emergency department committee wants to make a home study, the following brief outline is suggested:

A QUESTIONNAIRE FOR HOME USE

Facilities and Equipment

Is our emergency department so laid out that the doctors and nurses can give their best efforts?
Is it large enough for maximum loads?
Does it fit into our disaster plan?
Is it adequately equipped for conceivable emergencies?

Is the equipment in good condition and periodically inspected by those responsible for it?

Are the supplies and equipment well arranged?

Is everything labeled so it can be put into instant use?

Are all packaged sterile trays clearly labeled so that anyone may identify them?

Are x-ray and laboratory facilities available around the clock, including blood for transfusions?

Personnel

Is capable nursing service available immediately as needed? This means on the spot, or, if not, available from close at hand with the emergency department always having top priority?

Is medical staff coverage so planned as to provide maximum skills by the staff doctors?

Is a surgeon always on call or on standby status? Do these surgeons honor this responsibility?

Are there restrictions on staff privileges in the emergency department comparable to those elsewhere in the hospital?

Records

Are well-planned and usable record forms available?

Are these completed promptly and adequately?

Are they periodically audited?

General

Are we carrying out procedures that could be done better elsewhere in the hospital?

Does the medical staff review the scope and quality of care given in the emergency department periodically?

Do these reviews indicate consistent good care commensurate with staff experience and training?

Is the handling of injured patients within the hospital such as to prevent further damage?

Would administration and staff be satisfied with the quality of emergency department care if they or their families were the patients?

REFERENCES

1. Kennedy, R.H.: Our Fashionable Killer: Oration on trauma. *Bull Am Coll Surgeons,* 40:78–81, 1955.
2. Skudder, P.A., McCarroll, J.R., and Wade, P.A.: Hospital emergency facilities and services: A survey. *Bull Am Coll Surgeons,* 46:44–50, 1961.
3. Owens, J.C.: Survey discovers what is wrong with hospital emergency service. *Mod Hosp,* 106:82–85, 1966.

Chapter 20

MANUAL OF POLICIES AND PROCEDURES

Any emergency department should have a manual outlining the standard policies and procedures to be carried out. The physician members of the department committee will of necessity have to prepare most of this. There are sections, however, in which they will need consultation and advice from the nursing and administration departments. Indeed, some sections will be prepared by these departments. No one could write a manual that would be satisfactory in every hospital. It must be prepared locally.

The necessity for agreement by all concerned seems self-evident. This manual is not a specific guide to the practice of emergency department medicine. It is not an attempt to interfere with the judgment of the individual physician. It is, however, an attempt to keep emergency department procedures within certain commonly accepted boundaries. There is no field of medicine in which prompt and positive decisions are more often needed than in this department. There is no field in which the correct treatment will stand out more clearly and, by the same token, no field in which poor treatment will be so noticeable. This opens the hospital and doctor to the hazards of legal action. Most doctors will welcome guidelines approved by their confrères. If such guidelines are established by the staff and followed in the emergency department, the defense against negligence will usually not be difficult. This is particularly true if accurate and promptly written records are kept.

The size and detail covered by such a manual may vary greatly. Some hospitals have been able to reduce this to a few succinct pages, while others have prepared manuals of 50 or more pages. It is not wise to have this printed in permanent form, at least not the first edition. Practice will almost always call for revision, so a mimeographed policy manual will be best. Copies should be available for all staff members as well as residents and interns, in order that they may make themselves acquainted with its contents. Of course, a copy should be available in the department.

Rather than being a set of dogmatic directions regarding patient care, this manual, as usually drawn up, is more administrative in nature. It will thus avoid confusion, particularly among residents, interns, nurses, and others carrying various responsibilities in this department. Members of the attending staff will appreciate it, as it provides them with sound guidance and sometimes much-needed professional authority. Where it is decided to include specific treatment discussions, there should be general staff agreement on the principles involved. In highly departmentalized hospitals, it may be desirable to have the principles determined in departments and then approved by the staff.

In hospitals with house staffs, it may be decided to include in this manual specific instructions for care of certain injuries by interns and residents. Some of the thoughts presented in Chapter 15 regarding the care of wounds, fractures, and other conditions may be of value in planning these instructions. Except where the staff agrees on exact procedures, such as tetanus immunization, the instructions should always be written in such a way as to allow for the application of individual judgment. In the case of house officers, there may be a rule that approval by a member of the attending staff must be obtained if nonstandard procedures are to be followed.

Experience in preparing such a manual, and the opportunity to review those prepared in a number of hospitals, has suggested the following as items to be considered for inclusion.

Foreword

In this should be a brief statement of the purpose of the manual, making clear its limitations and restrictions as outlined in the foregoing.

Purpose of the Emergency Department

A concise statement of the purpose and function of this department should be included. This should be worded with care. On many occasions it will prove its worth, particularly if strangers question the attitudes of the personnel. If there is a notice posted in the department stating clearly the services it offers and the services it does not attempt to offer, this should agree exactly with the purpose of the department as stated in the manual. If the statement is changed in one of these places, the same change should be made in the other.

Responsibility

This should be clearly stated as belonging to a specifically named committee (the makeup of the committee need not be detailed), a department of the medical staff, the chief or chairman of a certain department, the hospital administrator, or whatever individual or group has been given this responsibility. This places authority where it belongs. Names of individuals should not be included as these will be subject to change.

Resident Staff

Rules and regulations outlining the responsibilities and limitations of residents and interns in hospitals having a house staff should be clearly stated. It should be made clear what they may do on their own responsibility and when they must consult a member of the attending staff. In accordance with prevailing rules and authority of members of the house staff as related to each other, in all departments of the hospital, there should be rules in the emergency department. For instance, certain procedures may call for approval of or supervision by the surgical or the medical resident.

Departmental Privileges

As pointed out in Chapter 7, "Staffing," members of the attending staff should not be allowed to carry out procedures in the emergency department for which they would not have privileges elsewhere in the hospital. This should be clearly stated in the policy manual.

Limitations on Procedures

When the staff agrees that certain procedures, i.e. repair of tendons or care of open fractures, should not be done in the emergency department, these limitations should be stated. It is just as important, however, to have a clear statement that in circumstances where delay would endanger a patient, they are authorized. It would not be possible to list all such circumstances, but a statement may be worded to cover them in general.

Duties of Personnel Other than Medical Staff

These may be listed in the form of a job description for each group involved. Daily, weekly, and monthly recurring duties should be noted. These would include such things as periodic reports, inspecting and servicing of equipment, and the replenishing of supplies. Where authority within each group or inter-group authority is involved, this should be made clear. Such outlines need not be worded so as to imply a distasteful relationship between groups, but rather to forestall misunderstandings regarding responsibilities.

Rules Affecting Personnel from Other Departments

These should be kept to a minimum. As stated in Chapter 9, every effort should be made to create and maintain a spirit of cooperation with other departments. There are, however, certain features that should be mentioned in this section of the policy manual. An example of these would be the matter of the removal of splints before the taking of x-rays. It should be clearly stated that no one other than the attending physician has the authority to authorize such removal.

Records

Copies of all record forms, including those used for requisitioning services from other departments, should be included in the manual. The responsibility for completing all forms, and a rule requiring prompt completion, should be included.

Release of Information Relating to Patients

This subject is discussed in Chapter 13, but specific statements of hospital policy should be in the manual.

Reporting of Certain Categories of Patients

State and local laws require notification of police, coroner, health authorities, or other representatives of the public under certain circumstances. These include such cases as communicable diseases, animal bites, poisonings, automobile accidents, murders, suicide, rape, or other indications of foul play. References to Health Department publications concerning these situations or laws or statutes requiring notification should be included in the manual.

Disposition of Specific Patients

Hospital policies concerning the admission or other disposition of certain classes of patients should be clearly stated. These would include various communicable diseases, psychotic patients, and others with regard to which each hospital usually has regulations. The care of psychotic patients is discussed by Drs. Branch and Worthylake in Chapter 17, but rules regarding their ultimate disposition might be included in the manual. A clear statement of the policies in the manual may prevent misunderstandings and even legal action. A statement concerning the management of unconscious patients is in order.

If standard procedure in the community calls for admission of certain categories of patients, such as veterans, military personnel, or public assistance patients, to other institutions, these procedures should be noted in the manual. There should be an index of the various health agencies in the community, with their telephone numbers, for use in advising patients or referring them.

D.O.A.'s and Deaths in the Department

Instructions regarding notification of the proper authorities and regarding disposition of bodies should be included. A cross-reference to the policy regarding release of news to the press is indicated here.

Anesthesia

Any rules applicable to the use of general anesthesia in the department should be noted. These would include preanesthetic requirements, such as a recorded history and physical examination, and record of laboratory tests.

Prophylaxis Against Infection

Immunization against tetanus should be outlined in accordance with staff agreement and any other appropriate references to prophylaxis included.

Asepsis

Rules requiring the wearing of caps and masks for certain procedures should be stated. Any rules or suggestions from the x-ray department should be included. Some admonition against the overuse of x-rays might be appropriate. Policies concerning prereduction and postreduction x-rays of fractures should be stated.

Patient Care Procedures

Without any attempt to prescribe treatment, the committee may decide to include in the policy manual references to specific procedures as reminders that they are accepted methods. Such reminders are particularly valuable in guiding new members of the house staff assigned to the department.

Consent for Anesthesia or Operation

A copy of the form to be used for this should be in the manual along with regulations as to its use. Procedures to be followed in the case of minors unaccompanied by parents, and, in the case of patients unable to sign a permit, should be stated. A valuable suggestion for summer camps or schools might be included to the effect that parents give written authority to camp or school officials to sign such consents.

Follow-up Care

Reminders regarding this are valuable from the standpoint of good care as well as legal responsibility. If a form is used for patients' instructions, a copy of this should be in the manual. This should include instructions regarding patients' own aftercare at home and reference to a specific physician or clinic.

The instructions should include warnings about reporting swelling, pain, fever, discharge, or anything else that might suggest complications.

Fees

When a fee schedule for various procedures has been adopted, this should be in the policy manual, as well as directions regarding the collection of fees. Unless the department is conducted as a free clinic, which not many are today, reference to the subject of physicians' fees should be included in the manual so that no patient will feel that he has discharged his obligation by paying the hospital fee.

Copies of all the insurance forms stocked in the department should be in the manual, so that personnel will know what forms to use in completing transactions involving insurance.

Education of Personnel in the Department

This subject is discussed in some detail in Chapter 18. If the department is used in the training program of residents or interns, it will be well to have this plan outlined. If there is a director of medical education, he may be the appropriate person to prepare this section of the manual.

Equipment and Its Care

There should be a list of all items of equipment, with the location indicated where movable items are to be kept when not in use. There should be instructions regarding the care, servicing, and replacement of such items. The responsibility for such care should be indicated.

Responsibility of On-call Physicians

The responsibilities of physicians assigned to the emergency department should be stated in the manual. This should include a clear statement regarding the answering of calls. There are valid objections to stating a time limit within which calls should be answered. Suppose a conscientious physician, who usually answered calls promptly, did not arrive within the specified time on a certain occasion. If for some reason the outcome of the treatment was not satisfactory, he might be held legally liable for this, although the time involved had not been an element in the poor result. On the other hand, any physician who answered his calls late as a routine should have this called to his attention and action taken if he did not improve his habits. The authority for dealing with such situations should be clearly designated as belonging to the chief of staff, department chief, or other officer of the medical staff.

Table of Contents

There should be a table of contents in the front of the manual so that time will not be lost in locating the section of interest. A complete index will be even more useful.

The operating of an emergency department without at least some written guidelines is like playing a game without rules. Hospitals that have spent time on the careful preparation of a *Manual of Policies and Procedures* have all found it valuable and many of them have revised it as experience indicated. That many hospitals have failed to prepare such a manual is indicated by Owens'* findings in Colorado. Only 12 of the 72 hospitals that he visited had one.

* Owens, J.C.: *Survey of Emergency Departments in Colorado.* A study under a Public Health Service grant, University of Colorado Medical Center, 1965.

Chapter 21

EMERGENCY DEPARTMENT
VS OUTPATIENT DEPARTMENT
Further Thoughts on Misuse and One Solution

Not many years ago, one of the pathways to full hospital staff membership was through the outpatient department. Whether seeing surgical outpatients and, after diagnosis, sending them into the hospital for someone else to operate on was adequate training for future surgical staff appointment might be open to question. When accompanied by preceptor training within the hospital, it probably gave the best background available to many young men before the widespread establishment of surgical residencies in the late thirties and since World War II.

The establishment of residencies has reduced the training activity in outpatient departments, but the activity has also been decreased by the attendance of fewer patients in these clinics. Outpatient hours have been decreased in many places. This may be one of the reasons why some of the patients who used to go there now go to the emergency department. At any rate, the influx of many nonemergency patients into the emergency departments has not been beneficial to these departments in preserving their real function.

The spread of insurance coverage through Blue Cross and Blue Shield as well as through commercial policies has no doubt reduced the percentage of patients needing free care or low pay care in the outpatient clinics, but this widespread insurance coverage has also channeled some of these policyholders into the emergency departments. Clauses in their insurance contracts have in some cases brought this about. A reevaluation of these insurance programs from all standpoints might lead to a rewriting of some of the policies to the benefit of all concerned. If patients are having their nonemergent medical needs classified as emergent because they are attended to in a department labeled "emergency," while it was not the intent of the policy to cover nonemergencies, then something is wrong.

If the health and accident insurance plans have been written so that payment will be made only when treatment is provided within the hospital building, with the idea that this will limit the payments to emergency cases, someone needs to talk to the carriers. Many people who show a minimum of initiative in bettering themselves from an income standpoint exhibit an amazing amount of resourcefulness in outwitting an insurance company. In this, the physician may become an unwitting accomplice. The demands by many unions for overall medical coverage in or out of hospital are well known. If someone is able to pay a realistic premium for such coverage, part of this emergency department problem may be solved. There are so many factors involved in this misuse of the department that it becomes evident that many interests should be represented in the solution. The insurance carriers might well have a part in it.

The provision of a facility for transient, one-visit patients without emergencies is one solution to the misuse of the emergency department. Emphasis need not be placed on speed in such a facility, but, as elsewhere in the hospital, quality of care is important. It is unreasonable to claim that nonemergent patients have the right to expect immediate attention if they go to a hospital instead of a doctor.

As described in Chapter 1, such plans as that in vogue at Yale–New Haven Hospital have shunted these patients into more appropriate channels, but that plan requires a resident staff, which most hospitals do not have. Difficult as it may seem in some communities to educate the public away from the emergency department when no emergency exists, it becomes much less difficult if there is some place to send them. It allows for placing some responsibility on the patient. It may be suggested to him that he call his own physician by telephone from the department, if he has not done so before coming. If he claims not to have one, he may be given a list of doctors from which to make a selection. Without his having been turned away, he is at least reminded that the hospital does not provide a doctor at all hours for patients not in acute distress. What to call this auxiliary facility, which is really for the convenience of the patients, is something that each hospital would have to decide, but it can serve the dual purpose of convenience to doctors and patients and relief of the emergency facilities. To fully exploit the advantages of such a facility, several things should be kept in mind:

1. It should be so separated from the emergency department that it will not be considered a subdivision of the latter. It need not be far removed physically but should, if possible, have a separate entrance, or at least a separate directional approach after a patient has come in from the outside.

2. It should have a name that makes it stand apart from the emergency department in thinking and discussion, as well as in fact.

3. It should have a separate record system with different record forms.

4. Nurse staffing need not be constant, but it should be distinct from that of the emergency department, unless the hospital personnel is so limited as to make this impractical.

5. It does not need constant physician staffing, for its main function is to provide facilities for the members of the medical staff to treat patients without going to their private offices. A meeting of patient and physician here may be initiated by either party.

If there is an organized and equipped outpatient department, it may take the place of this auxiliary facility, even in off hours.

One of its greatest values is that it simplifies the explanation to the public, that the emergency department is for *emergencies only*. Such an auxiliary facility answers the charge that the hospital is not prepared to take care of the medical needs of the community, yet at the same time it acts as a reminder to the patient that what he really needs is a doctor—not a building, and that he might save time and trouble, not to mention expense, if he would get one.

This facility will provide for minor outpatient operations, which procedures have been known to tie up badly needed emergency rooms. Nothing can be more frustrating to an emergency department nurse or to the physician on call than to have the major portion of the department occupied with a half-finished minor operation when several injured patients badly in need of care arrive at the entrance.

Another reason for keeping nonemergent minor surgical procedures out of the emergency department is the incidence of frank infection among these cases. "Incision and drainage of abscess" is a frequently scheduled outpatient operation. This is not a good procedure to do in a room or on stretchers where open fractures or other wounds may be treated soon afterward. There is time to clean the room in the nonemergency facility before other patients are admitted.

This adjunct facility is not a new idea. It was known as the Consultation Department in the hospital where I took my residency. This would seem to be an appropriate name. We simply called it "Consultation" for short. This was in a 600-bed hospital, yet this department had merely a skeleton staff because nothing of an urgent nature took place there. In fact, some of the attending physicians and surgeons had nurses or secretaries in their own employ meet them there after lunch so that patients might be seen before the doctors went to their outside offices. This department was available at any time with facilities for examinations, surgical dressings, and other such procedures. The emergency department was kept free for emergencies.

The convenience of this department both to patients and physicians as well as its educational value in keeping nonemergencies out of the emergency department are sufficient to warrant its establishment if space is available. As stated above, an outpatient department may be used in the same way for either private or medically indigent patients.

Chapter 22

LEGAL ASPECTS OF THE EMERGENCY DEPARTMENT

Arthur F. Southwick, Jr.

INTRODUCTION

Ordinarily, a patient does not have a legal right to be admitted formally to either a private, voluntary, or governmental hospital or to be seen and treated, for example, in an outpatient clinic. This is to say that as a general rule there is no common law or statutory duty on the part of the hospital to serve all who apply for accommodation or service, and as a general rule there has been no imposition of a duty to serve by statutory law.

With respect, however, to some hospitals owned and operated by government in some jurisdictions, the statutes may be construed as creating a right to be served and/or admitted in certain classes of individuals. Statutes creating certain governmental hospitals and specifying the purposes to be accomplished by the hospital may define or designate groups or classes of persons to be served as, for example, the population of a given county or patients diagnosed as suffering a particular disease. A review of such statutes and an interpretation of the extent of the legal right to be admitted as a patient is well beyond the scope of this chapter on the legal aspects of emergency care.*

Also, the general rule denying a legal right in the patient to be admitted may be changed in circumstances where the hospital has voluntarily undertaken by contract an obligation to serve. Such a contract could be between the hospital and an identifiable

* See generally, *Hospital Law Manual*, Admitting and Discharge. Pittsburgh, Aspen Systems Corporation.

321

class or group of patients or between the hospital and, for example, an employer, with the latter's employees designated as beneficiaries of the undertaking.* Naturally and understandably, an obligation created by an express contract must be performed.

Both of the above exceptions or modifications of the general concept that a hospital has no duty to serve or formally admit patients are quite limited in application and effect. Neither apply in most situations or in the vast majority of the nation's communities. Accordingly, in 1971, the general rule of law is under attack from at least two specific directions, both of which could have a profound effect upon traditional and historical hospital policies and also upon medical staff organization.

The first attack on the rule of nonduty to serve arises as a result of the Hill-Burton Hospital Act which, it is alleged in several lawsuits currently pending, requires participating hospitals to provide a "reasonable volume" of free care or at least provide services below cost to those patients unable to pay. The aim of the suits is to establish that low-income patients have a right to be served by the local, community hospital which has received Hill-Burton funding, and that, accordingly, hospital policy requiring evidence of ability to pay prior to admission is in violation of the Hill-Burton legislation. Also, it is alleged that such policy violates the due process and equal protection clauses of the 14th Amendment to the Federal Constitution. The resolution of these issues must await, of course, final determination of the currently pending suits.†

---

* *Norwood Hospital v. Howton*, 32 Ala. App. 375, 26 So.2d 427 (1946).

† One of these pending suits is entitled *Euresti v. Stenner*, Federal District Court, Colorado. The relevant Hill-Burton provision is 42 U.S.C., Section 291 (c) (e); the regulation promulgated by the Surgeon General is 42 CFR, Sec. 53.111. The latter in effect requires the facility receiving construction funds to give assurance that it will furnish a "reasonable volume of services to persons unable to pay therefore." In the *Euresti* case, the court in May 1971 dismissed the suit on the basis that the legislation did not create a contract between the United States and defendant hospitals and that the plaintiffs as private citizens have no right or standing to sue. The decision has been appealed. On the issue of whether the legislation impliedly gives a private cause of action a contrary decision has been reached in *Cook v. Ochsner Foundation Hospital*, 319 F. Supp. 603 (E.D. La. 1970), relying on *Gomez v. Florida Employment Service*, 417 F2d 569 (5th Circuit 1969).

The second attack on the rule of nonduty comes through, or arises from, the maintenance and operation of the hospital's emergency department. This is the subject matter of this chapter. It is perfectly evident that the American public expects service from the nation's hospitals and their medical staffs. Primarily, through the mechanism of the private lawsuit, judicial decision is establishing a duty on the part of the hospital's emergency facility to at least see and treat or refer all patients who apply for service. Accordingly, hospitals and their staffs must be organized and prepared to meet the expectations of the public as expressed in the judicial decisions reviewed henceforth. The most recent decisions of influential courts would appear consistent with the newly developed and frequently articulated philosophy that health care is a right and not a privilege.

HOSPITAL EMERGENCY CARE AND TREATMENT

Factual Situation and Legal Issues

Considered here are those situations where a patient presents himself at the hospital, usually at the emergency department or facility, requesting examination and treatment. Frequently, such a person will appear without benefit of a private physician who is a member of the hospital's medical staff or will appear at a time when his private physician is unavailable. The hospital's legal responsibilities to the patient may depend upon, first, whether the situation is governed by statutory or common law; secondly whether the institution in fact has an emergency department; and finally, the apparent condition of the patient at the time he presents himself for diagnosis, advice, and treatment.

Initially, the question is whether or not a hospital must maintain an emergency care facility. If it must or if it voluntarily maintains a facility, the issue then becomes one of the extent of the institution's duty to the patient.

Necessity for the Maintenance of Emergency Care Facilities

The common law does not impose a duty upon a general community hospital to provide for the treatment and care of emergency patients. This means then that a hospital, governmental or private, generally need not have any special room, equipment, or personnel for the care of those who suddenly fall ill or who are the victims of accident.

In some jurisdictions, however, there are statutory requirements mandating either directly or indirectly the maintenance of emergency care facilities for certain types or categories of hospitals. In Wisconsin, for example, there is a statute requiring county hospitals located in counties having a population of 250,000 or more "to establish and maintain . . . an emergency unit or department for the treatment . . . of persons in said county who may meet with accidents or be suddenly afflicted with illness not contagious."* Not only then is there a duty to maintain an emergency facility, there is a duty to treat such persons, although the statute authorizes in effect "safe removal" of the patient to another hospital or to his home and thus does not require formal admission of all such patients. Moreover, the statute permits the county to provide this emergency care by contract with a private hospital. The point is that the statute casts upon local county government the obligation to provide emergency care facilities either directly or by contract.

In Illinois, a statute applicable to both private and governmental hospitals where surgical operations are performed requires the hospital to extend emergency care.† Pennsylvania requires all hospitals receiving payments for care of indigents to have at least one licensed doctor or intern on call at all times.‡ New York provides that operating certificates can be revoked for any general hospital that refuses to provide emergency care.§ In practical effect, then, such statutes as these, which attempt to assure that emergency care will be available, require the establishment of and maintenance of an emergency department. Violation will be penalized as provided for in the particular statute, perhaps a criminal sanction. Moreover, and more significant perhaps than the usual criminal sanction, violation of such a statute could be the basis of a private civil law suit for damages.

* Wisconsin Stat. Ann., Section 46.21(8) (b).
† Illinois Stat. Ann., Title 111½, Section 86 and 87 (Smith-Hurd 1966).
‡ Pa. Stat. Ann., Title 35, Section 435 (1964).
§ N.Y. Publ. Health Law, Section 2806.

It is suggested that these statutes represent a trend toward requiring hospitals to establish and maintain emergency care facilities and staff. The public expects community, general hospitals to be so equipped. The trend will have to be monitored and coordinated with sound public policy pertaining to area-wide planning of hospital facilities and services. Granted the fact that every community and every population group should have ready and convenient access to a hospital emergency department, it does not follow that all general hospitals should be legally required to maintain relatively expensive emergency care capabilities. *

Duty to Treat and Aid

At common law, there is no duty to aid another in peril. This doctrine, even though contrary to the morals and the ethics of the medical profession, has been applied to physicians and to hospitals as well as to lay persons. Hence, a physician has no common law responsibility to respond to a call for help from one not already his patient or from a person acting on behalf of one not his patient.† Similarly, a hospital, if it voluntarily without legal compulsion maintains an emergency care department, need

---

* In 1970, the Illinois State Hospital Licensing Board approved regulations, consistent with the statute previously cited, allowing hospitals to pool their emergency care facilities and staff. The regulations recognize three levels of service: "comprehensive," "basic," and "standby."

† Illustrative is the case of *Childs v. Weis,* 440 S.W.2d 104 (Texas App. 1969). A pregnant patient presented herself at the hospital emergency room at 2 A.M., apparently suffering from bleeding and thinking herself to be in labor. The nurse on duty conducted an examination and telephoned the staff physician on call. The doctor, a private practitioner, told the nurse to tell the patient to telephone her private physician for advice. The hospital as a matter of policy did not require the physician on call to see and examine all emergency room patients. The nurse apparently misrelayed the message and told the patient to proceed to see her private doctor, located some miles away. After leaving the hospital and while enroute, the baby was born and lived but twelve hours. In a suit against the physician, the court held that a dismissal of the action was proper on the basis that the doctor's duty to exercise reasonable care was dependent upon a contract with the patient and that here there was no such contract and, hence, no duty to treat. In other words, no doctor-patient relationship had been established and, accordingly, the physician was not liable for even an arbitrary refusal to respond to the call. Moreover, he was not liable for the negligence of the nurse, if any, since she was not his employee. Suit was not brought against the hospital.

not by application of the early common law, employ its facilities and staff to aid the person who presents himself for treatment. Recent cases, however, strongly suggest that this judicial attitude is changing, at least with respect to hospitals which maintain emergency care facilities, simply because the public expects aid and sound moral doctrine dictates that aid be extended where capabilities are present. These cases will be reviewed.

The only common law exception to the rule that there is no duty to aid another in peril is when the conduct of the one failing to aid was responsible for the victim being in peril. In such circumstances, failing to aid could result in liability. Some cases, however, restricted liability to negligent conduct which placed the plaintiff in peril. In short, the plaintiff to recover had to show first, that *negligent* conduct of the defendant placed him in peril; and second, that the defendant then failed in his duty to aid. Other cases have found liability for failure to aid whenever any type of conduct on the part of the defendant put the plaintiff in a position of peril.

This common law exception, however, has practically no application to hospitals in the context of this discussion because normally the hospital would not act in such a way to place one not a current hospitalized patient or visitor in peril. The usual situation is simply that a person seeking aid presents himself at the hospital. The question then is whether there is any legal duty on the part of the hospital to serve such a person.

The traditional common law answer would be in the negative. However, in the first place, statutory law in particular jurisdictions may directly or by inference change the common law. Statutes in Wisconsin, Illinois, New York, and Pennsylvania, for example, were noted in the preceding section discussing requirements for the establishment of emergency care facilities. Also to be noted, is a Florida statute pertaining to certain governmental hospitals which are declared to be for the benefit of those who fall ill or are the victims of accidents within the governmental boundaries.* From statutory language mandating the maintenance of emergency care facilities, it is reasonable to infer a duty to aid victims of an emergency. An affirmative duty to

---

* Florida Stat. Ann., Section 155.16 (1943).

aid follows logically from a duty to maintain emergency care facilities.

More express and direct on the issue of a duty to aid is a relatively new statute in California. The act, passed in 1970, requires that hospitals having "appropriate facilities and qualified personnel" provide emergency care in cases of serious injury or illness. The law further provides that the hospital, its personnel, and the physician are not liable in damages for refusal to render emergency care, if good faith and reasonable care were exercised in determining the appropriateness of the available facilities and personnel to care for the patient.*

Certainly, it is clear that a public hospital or a private hospital receiving Hill-Burton funds or other governmental support may not refuse emergency care or hospital admission on the basis of race, color, creed, or national origin. To do so would clearly violate the Fourteenth Amendment to the Federal Constitution.†

Judicial law, moreover, is developing a duty to aid under certain circumstances and, accordingly, the traditional common law response to the question posed above is no longer a reliable guide to hospitals. In the recent case of *Williams v. Hospital Authority of Hall County,* the Georgia Appellate Court held that a governmental hospital which has an emergency care department must extend aid to the victim of an accident who had presented himself at the hospital for treatment of a fracture.‡ The court stressed that the defendant hospital was tax supported and a public institution, and expressly rejected the argument that the hospital had an absolute right to refuse emergency services. The judge described a refusal to serve where an emergency care facility was available as "repugnant." Although the decision was carefully limited in applicability to a governmental hospital, it would be a short step indeed to extend this same philosophy to a voluntary hospital which maintains an emergency department.

---

* California Health and Safety Code Ann., Section 1407.5 (Supp. 1970).
† *Simkins v. Moses H. Cone Memorial Hospital,* 323 F.2d 959 (1963); *Flagler Hospital v. Hayling,* 344 F.2d 950 (1964); *Eaton v. Grubbs,* 329 F.2d 710 (1964).
‡ 119 Ga. App. 626 (1969); 168 S.E.2d 336.

The Missouri Supreme Court has apparently already done so. In *Stanturf v. Sipes*, a patient with frozen feet was refused treatment and admission to a private hospital for the reason that initially he was not able to pay an advance cash deposit, and the refusal was continued even after friends offered the deposit, apparently on the basis that further payment could not be assured. The delay in care resulted in amputation of both feet. The court set forth an opinion to the effect that a hospital which has an emergency service holds itself out as providing care and may not then refuse.* Hence, even if a preadmission cash deposit requirement is legally justifiable for a nonemergency patient, it is not justifiable with respect to the patient who presents himself in need of immediate care. It is suggested that the holding of this court should now be accepted as the rule governing hospital emergency room policies.

Prior to the *Williams* and *Sipes* cases, the Delaware court had issued a landmark decision in *Wilmington General Hospital v. Manlove.*† When the family pediatrician could not be located, the mother of an infant took the child to the hospital emergency department. The patient was suffering from acute diarrhea and high temperature. The nurse on duty refused to examine the baby or call another doctor, on the basis that the patient was already under the care of a private physician. She did try to call the private doctor but was unsuccessful and then suggested that if he still couldn't be reached the mother return with the infant to the hospital clinic the next day. The patient died at home four hours later. In a suit for damages, the hospital was held liable on the basis that the nurse at least had a duty to determine whether an "unmistakable" emergency existed and, if so, to extend aid. Hence, as a minimum, the nurse in the emergency department must exercise reasonable care to ascertain the patient's condition and then act accordingly. A professional judgment made with reasonable care under all the facts and circumstances to the effect that the patient was not in need of immediate medical care and treatment would not result in liability under the *Manlove* reasoning. Nevertheless, since it is normally beyond the scope

* 447 S.W.2d 558; 35 A.L.R.3rd 834 (1969).
† 54 Del. 15, 174 A.2d 135 (1961).

of nursing practice to make a medical diagnosis, it is difficult to see how a nurse can adequately perform her duty and protect the hospital from possible liability unless she calls a licensed physician to examine the patient and recommend treatment.

Hence, on the basis of these judicial decisions, it is strongly recommended that hospital policy require that all patients presenting themselves at the emergency department be seen, examined, and advised by a licensed physician. The physician, then, in the exercise of his professional judgment orders formal admission, transfer to another institution, or return to home. Diagnosis and advice by telephone is not recommended, as it is legally possible to create a physician-patient or hospital-patient relationship by telephone and, accordingly, create a duty to exercise reasonable care and skill under all the circumstances. There is risk of breach of this duty when diagnosis by telephone is relied upon, especially when the doctor does not personally know the patient and his condition.*

The foregoing recommendation is also based upon the long-standing and well-accepted common law rule that the voluntary beginning of aid creates a duty to exercise reasonable care under all the facts and circumstances. The rule clearly applies to both physicians and hospitals. The slightest act of aid or exercise of control over the patient may be legally the starting of aid, thereby bringing into play this judicial doctrine. To illustrate, in *Bourgeois v. Dade County* the police brought an unconscious patient to the hospital. The physician on emergency call duty conducted only a cursory examination without benefit of x-rays, decided that the patient was intoxicated, and approved removal of the patient to jail. There he died, and it was then established that the patient had been suffering from broken ribs which had punctured the chest.† The issue of negligence was one for jury determination.

There are many other cases involving the same principles and the finding of liability for negligence. No attempt is made here to call attention to all of these decisions. However, in addition to *Bourgeois,* there are other important cases that a hospital

---

* Compare the case of *Childs v. Weis,* 440 S.W.2d 104 (Texas App. 1969).
† 99 So.2d 575; 72 A.L.R.2d 391 (1957).

administrator should be familiar with, namely, *New Biloxi Hospital v. Frazier,* Jones v. City of New York,† Methodist Hospital v. Ball,‡ and O'Neill v. Montefiore Hospital.§* In *Frazier, Jones,* and *Ball,* the facts were fundamentally the same. In all instances, the victims of violence or accident were accepted into the emergency department, and hospital staff failed to exercise reasonable care in diagnosis, treatment, and disposition of the case. In the *Jones* case, an intern of a voluntary hospital cleaned and dressed stab wounds and, without further care, ordered the patient transferred to a city hospital, the delay causing death. In both *Frazier* and *Ball,* the patients were unattended for a considerable length of time (45 minutes in the *Ball* case; 2 hours in *Frazier*), with minimal attention and diagnosis from hospital nursing and medical staff, and then transferred to other institutions, with adverse results. These cases emphasize the legal and humane necessity of exercising reasonable care in making a diagnosis and deciding the course (and place) of treatment.‖ The litigated cases also show the necessity for hospital personnel to determine which patients need immediate attention. Delay cannot be excused on the basis that others are being attended. Of course, to collect damages, it is required that the plaintiff prove, usually by expert witness testimony, that the delay in diagnosis and treatment or the delay occasioned by the transfer to another institution was the proximate cause of death or worsened condition.°

The *O'Neill* case in New York is one of the most instructive of all. A man and his wife arrived at the hospital emergency department in the early morning hours, stating to the nurse on duty that they believed he was experiencing a heart attack. Upon inquiry the patient revealed that he was a participant in

* 245 Miss. 185; 146 So.2d 882 (1962).
† 134 N.Y.S.2d 779 (1954).
‡ 50 Tenn. App. 460; 362 S.W.2d 475 (1961).
§ 202 N.Y.S.2d 436 (1960).
‖ For still another case involving an inadequate examination and a decision by a hospital intern in the emergency room to send the patient home before the results of a throat culture were known, see *Barcia v. Society of N.Y. Hospital,* 241 N.Y.S.2d 373 (1963).
° *Ruvio v. North Broward Hospital District,* 186 So.2d 45 (Florida 1966), affirmed 195 So.2d 567.

the Health Insurance Plan of New York. The nurse thereupon informed the O'Neill's that the hospital did not serve such individuals and that it would be necessary for the patient to see his H.I.P. physician. The hospital nurse did, however, telephone the H.I.P. physician, and, in a conversation directly with the patient, the physician apparently told him to return home and that he could be seen at Plan facilities later in the day. The hospital nurse thereupon refused a further request for examination by a staff member at defendant hospital. The patient returned home and died before he could see his physician.

The court held that there were two issues to be resolved by a jury. First, did the nurse's action in telephoning the H.I.P. physician constitute the beginning of aid, thus creating the duty to exercise reasonable care? Secondly, if the first issue is answered in the affirmative, did the nurse exercise the proper standard of care? With respect to the first question, it might normally be expected that juries will not be sympathetic to the hospital. In other words, even in a jurisdiction which nominally recognizes the historical common law rule that there is no duty to aid one who presents himself at the hospital, the slightest act by emergency department personnel on behalf of the patient is likely to be interpreted as the exercise of control, thus creating a duty to act reasonably.

In logic, of course, the issues emphasized in the *O'Neill* and similar cases decided in the early 1960's and prior thereto are now moot in the light of the *Manlove, Williams,* and *Sipes* cases. In other words, if there is a positive duty on the part of a hospital having an emergency department to recognize a medical emergency or simply to extend aid to all who present themselves, it is not necessary to argue or determine whether aid was in fact started or control over the patient exercised. By either process of reasoning, however, the proper conduct is clear—all patients who present themselves should be seen, examined, and treated as their condition requires.*

Obviously, this does not mean that all emergency department patients must be formally admitted to the hospital. The duty is

* See generally, Powers, *Hospital Emergency Service and the Open Door,* 66 *Michigan Law Review* 1455, No. 7, May, 1968.

to exercise reasonable care under all the facts and circumstances. Hence, transfer to another hospital is justified when no negligence occurs in diagnosis or treatment rendered in the emergency department, and when the exercise of reasonable professional judgment determines that the transfer will not aggravate or worsen the patient's condition. Such was the situation in the recent case of *Joyner v. Alton Ochsner Medical Foundation,* where an accident victim was properly cared for on an emergency first-aid basis as his condition required in accordance with recognized standards of medical care and then transferred to another hospital with the approval of his wife when they were unable to pay the required deposit for admission.* The case is clearly distinguishable from the *Sipes* litigation in the Missouri court previously discussed because in that situation all care was refused, even after third parties agreed to pay the deposit.

Similarly, the rendition of emergency care does not obligate a hospital to violate its legitimate rules regarding formal admission, or commit it to admit patients that it is not adequately equipped to treat on a continuing basis. In *Birmingham Baptist Hospital v. Crews,* a relatively old case, the hospital had a rule that patients with contagious disease could not be admitted. A victim of diphtheria was seen and treated in the emergency department. She expired soon after being sent home. The court held that the hospital could not be held liable, saying that there was no legal right to formal admission, that requiring the hospital in this instance to violate its rule regarding contagious disease would encourage the hospital to refuse even emergency aid in the future, and that requiring admission might endanger the health of other patients.†

In summary, patients who present themselves at the hospital emergency department should never be turned away until seen and examined by a licensed physician who determines the seriousness of the illness or injury and then orders admission, return home, or referral to another facility, depending upon the facts and circumstances of each particular case. Undue de-

* 230 So.2d 913 (Louisiana 1970).
† 229 Ala. 398, 157 So.224 (1934).

lays should not be tolerated. These policies should be expressed in clearly understood, written rules which are readily capable of implementation by hospital personnel and emergency department physicians. Written rules which are subsequently ignored or violated could be evidence of negligence; hence, it is extremely important to follow established hospital policies which are expressed in written form.

It is also important to fully implement and follow standards of emergency care promulgated by both public and private agencies or professional groups. An example of the former is rules and regulations promulgated by the state department or agency responsible under law for hospital licensure. If there is a licensure law in the particular state and if there are regulations pertaining to emergency care, a violation of said regulations could be evidence of negligence in a civil suit by the patient for damages. Most important, further, is the fact that standards of private agencies, such as the Joint Commission on Accreditation of Hospitals and the American College of Surgeons, have the same legal implications. Both groups have published standards relative to emergency department equipment, staffing, and the rendition of care. For example, the Joint Commission's *Standards for Emergency Services* states the principle as follows: "Adequate appraisal and advice or initial treatment shall be rendered to any ill or injured person who presents himself at the hospital."* Under this principle, Standard I requires a well-defined plan for providing care consistent with community need and the capability of the hospital. The interpretations reveal that this does not mean that all hospitals must actually maintain a full-service emergency department. Rather, the plan for emergency care may recognize limited capabilities or even may recognize that all emergency patients may be transferred to other institutions. The major point is that a plan for emergency care must exist, and if the hospital does in fact have the means for care of the patient, he should not be arbitrarily sent elsewhere. If, then, an emergency department is maintained, further standards relate to or-

* *Standards for Accreditation of Hospitals,* Joint Commission on Accreditation of Hospitals, October 1969, p. 45.

ganization, direction, staffing, facilities, the existence of written policies, and the maintenance of medical records.

It also should be noted that the Medicare *Conditions of Participation* contain standards for emergency care. They are similar to those promulgated by the Joint Commission on Accreditation.

The major legal point to be emphasized here is that regulations of public or governmental agencies and standards of private agencies—together with hospital rules often expressed in medical staff bylaws—are introducable into evidence for jury consideration in a liability suit for damages.*

Also to be stressed is the necessity to maintain written medical records for each person seen in the emergency room, even if that person is not formally admitted to the hospital. Such records are of course mandatory in the interests of adequate patient care. Moreover, the hospital may be called upon later to document in the courtroom the standards of care rendered to a particular patient, in which event a medical chart is indispensable. Included should be the instructions given the patient for continuing care should he be sent home, or information furnished an institution or physician to whom he is referred.

All of the foregoing cases and discussion of hospital liability arising out of the emergency department situation must be qualified by the doctrine of governmental immunity from tort liability in any case involving a state or local governmental hospital. Immunity of the state and its agencies from suit is a matter of individual state law. Also, in one or two states which still retain the remnants of charitable immunity, the outcome of a suit for damages against a charitable hospital would be controlled by the doctrine. But, of course, notions of hospital immunity for tort never protect the individual emergency department nurse, technician, or physician from individual liability. Moreover, by virtue of the Federal Tort Claims Act, a hospital owned and operated by the federal government is fully liable in tort to the same extent as a private hospital.

---

* *Darling v. Charleston Community Memorial Hospital,* 33 Ill.2d 326, 211 N.E.2d 253, (1965).

STAFFING THE EMERGENCY DEPARTMENT

All of the foregoing suggests that the legal duty of reasonable care owed patients presenting themselves at the emergency department mandates that the department be well organized, staffed with qualified personnel, and be possessed of necessary equipment and facilities to assure prompt diagnosis and treatment.

Organizationally, the department must be an integral part of the medical staff and accountable to relevant staff committees for the quality of care. Ultimately, the governing body of the hospital is responsible for the professional standards of the emergency department just as the board is responsible for all other clinical work in the institution.* Medical staff privileges in the emergency department should be delineated on an individual basis for the physicians staffing the facility as is done in other hospital departments.

For moderately sized and larger hospitals, staffing of the emergency department with nurses and interns supported by medical staff serving on a rotating on-call basis is no longer satisfactory to meet the expectations of the public and to perform the legal responsibilities required in the malpractice cases. Where physician coverage is limited to an on-call basis, there is too much opportunity for error in diagnosis and/or delay in treatment which leads directly to unfortunate situations and accelerates the liability problems illustrated by the cases reviewed previously. Prospects for liability may, perhaps ironically, be enhanced by the modern specialization of medical practice. This is to say that some specialists may, in fact, not be competent to deal with certain emergency cases and hence should not be on emergency duty. Clearly, substantial efforts must yet be made in many hospitals to correct what is probably the weakest link in standards of medical care provided the community.

Hence, hospitals called upon in their respective communities to furnish full-scale emergency services should have the facility staffed on a full-time basis by licensed, experienced phy-

Ibid.

sicians. Recognition of emergency medicine as a specialty might well facilitate and encourage further development of full-time arrangements.

Hospitals have several alternatives available to accomplish full-time physician coverage of the emergency department. In most states, the nonprofit institution may employ physicians directly on salary. This is to say that the judicial rule prohibiting a corporation from practicing medicine will not inhibit or prevent salaried arrangements. The rule was announced in some cases years ago to discourage commercialization and exploitation of the professional person and to emphasize that the physician owes his individual loyalties to his patient. However, the rule was developed in the context of the private, profit-making corporation and is believed to have little or no relevance to the modern voluntary hospital.

More typical than the direct employment of salaried physicians for emergency department staff is a contractual arrangement with a corporation of physicians or a partnership, whereby the physicians undertake to provide full-time coverage. Nearly all states now permit professional individuals to incorporate their practice under authority granted by special statute. Such a contract must be carefully drafted to obligate adequately the corporation or partnership to provide the services contemplated by the hospital and yet retain for the hospital adequate control with respect to privileges of the emergency department physicians and the standards of their practice. By entering into such an arrangement, the hospital must not abdicate its ultimate responsibilities for one quality of patient care. The contract, among other provisions, must provide guidelines for the following responsibilities: the supervision of hospital nurses and house staff, equipment and facilities, fees and billing, and the referral of patients. Also, the document must provide for the term of the arrangement and renewal. Above all, the medical staff of the hospital must be involved in monitoring the standards of practice in the emergency service, even when that service is contracted to an "independent" group of physicians.

The financial arrangements between hospital and the group of physicians may legally consist of two charges to the patient—

one for hospital services and another for the physician's service. The physician group may bill directly to the patient or may assign the account to the hospital for collection. Moreover, the hospital may legally guarantee the physicians an agreed-upon annual or periodic minimum income.

When the hospital contracts for emergency department coverage in the above fashion with a corporation or partnership of physicians, a legal question arises with respect to hospital liability for the malpractice or negligence of one of the doctors. The contract will normally recite that the physicians are "independent contractors," and at common law under the doctrine of *respondeat superior,* an employer is not legally liable for the negligence or other tort of an independent contractor. The reason given for this long-established rule is that an employer has no right to control the means and methods of the independent contractor's work, although the employer does control ultimately the overall specifications and quality of the contractor's performance.

The Georgia Appellate Court adhered to this traditional legal concept to hold in 1969 that the hospital was not liable for the negligence of a physician staffing the emergency department.* Said doctor was a member of a medical partnership under contract with the hospital. The court observed that the hospital retained no control over individual, professional decisions of the physicians, and the contract recited that they were considered to be independent contractors. Identification of the partnership's general responsibilities and surveillance of standards of practice by the medical staff was not sufficient "control" to deny the hospital the defense of independent contractor.

A contrary result has been reached by the Supreme Court of Delaware. Even if a physician is an independent contractor vis-à-vis the hospital, the hospital can be held liable for the negligence of the doctor if the institution has "held out" or "represented" to the patient that the doctor is its agent or employee. This is the doctrine of Apparent Agency and,

---

* *Pogue v. Hospital Authority of DeKalb County,* 120 Ga. App. 230, 170 S.E.2d 53 (1969).

when applied, justifies the imposition of liability on the hospital for the wrong of one not in fact its employee. In *Vanaman v. Milford Memorial Hospital, Inc.*, the patient appeared at the emergency department having twisted her ankle in an accident. The family physician was not available; the patient and her mother indicated no preference with respect to choice of physician. Thereupon, the staff doctor on call was summoned, and his treatment resulted in injury to the patient. The trial court dismissed the suit against the hospital on the general basis that the institution had not held itself out as a "provider of medical care." On appeal, however, the Supreme Court reversed, saying that it was a question for the jury whether the patient was referred to the doctor acting in his private capacity or, in the alternate, whether the doctor was staffing the emergency department as agent of the hospital.° The fact that the physician was not paid directly by the hospital is relevant but not conclusive.

It is evident, of course, that not all hospitals are able to provide full-time physician presence in the emergency department or even provide 24-hour physician on-call coverage. From a legal point of view, such hospitals providing limited emergency service should make their limitations clear in a tactful manner to their respective communities. The institution should not give the impression of full-service capabilities when such is not the case.

In metropolitan and suburban areas having several hospitals with overlapping service areas, not all of these institutions should undertake, or represent that they undertake, full emergency service. In short, regional planning and rationalization of facilities and services is needed. This must be done on a voluntary basis that is truly effective or perhaps by statutory health facility planning laws. Some hospitals, perhaps, should have no emergency facility, others should have limited capabilities, and still others should have full service and permanent staffing.

° 272 A.2d 718 (Delaware 1970). Cases with similar reasoning are *Lundberg v. Bay View Hospital*, 175 Ohio State 133, 191 N.E.2d 821 (1963), involving a pathologist, and *Kober v. Stewart*, 148 Mont. 117, 417 P.2d 476 (1966), involving radiologists.

After the development and implementation of such regional plans, the public in general and police agencies and ambulance companies in particular should be made aware of each hospital's capability for the rendition of emergency care. Not only is such regional planning necessary as a matter of economics of health care, it is necessary as a matter of quality of care. Enhancement in the level of quality of care on a community basis will certainly have a favorable impact upon the legal problems currently facing hospital emergency departments.

Chapter 23

QUESTIONS AND ANSWERS

O ver the last twelve or thirteen years it has been my privilege to participate in a number of programs dealing with emergency medical care all the way from Boston to Seattle. In some of these I have read formal papers, but many of them have been panel discussions or open forums allowing questions from the audience. As moderator or panelist, I have accumulated a number of questions. It seems appropriate to ask some of these questions again here and answer them. The following is only a partial list of these sessions where questions were asked, and it is presented by listing the sponsoring organizations to indicate the types of audiences in attendance. These included physicians, nurses, hospital administrators and trustees, first-aid workers, ambulance crews, and even law enforcement officers.

New England Hospital Assembly
St. Barnabas Hospital (Livingston, New Jersey)
Ohio State Medical Association
Illinois Hospital Association and Illinois Medical Society
Academy of Medicine of New Jersey
New Jersey Committee on Trauma
Chicago Heart Association
Chicago Press Club
Cook County Association of Hospital Administrators
Chicago Medical Society
Shelby County (Tennessee) Medical Society
North Carolina Chapter, American College of Surgeons
Idaho Hospital Association
Washington State Medical Association

These questions have been selected because they have more than local interest.

Q: *Are emergency services in American hospitals as poor as some lay writers would have the public believe?*

A: No. Definitely not, and in spite of, not because of, the stories in the lay press, they are improving. It is astounding what editors of newspapers and magazines will accept from their staff and free-lance writers and publish as news. In some cases, the authors have pointed out in a constructive way things that the public should know, but far too often they have been written in a sensational manner, twisting the facts, telling half truths and doing nothing but break down the confidence of the public in hospitals trying to serve the public. A recent example is an article entitled, "Curing the Emergency Room."[1] Its title, with the emphasis on improvement, leaves the reader disappointed. The writer makes enough erroneous statements to immediately disqualify himself as knowledgeable, much less an authority. For instance, he states, "Most hospitals use interns to man their emergency rooms today." No more than 20 percent of hospitals in the United States have interns, so most could not, even if they wanted to, staff them with interns. In many cases where interns do work in emergency departments, they are under the supervision of more experienced doctors. This writer is describing conditions as they were a number of years ago. He implies that the practice of hiring "unlicensed foreign physicians" to man emergency departments is widespread. This again is not true. It is true that many foreign educated physicians do work in emergency departments in this country, but a great many of them are licensed in the states where they work. If not, they have passed the E.C.F.M.G. examination, which is more difficult than many state board examinations. Some of the best emergency department doctors I have known were foreign born and graduates of foreign medical schools.

This author also speaks of an organization of emergency department physicians that does not exist and fails to mention either of the two that do exist. He writes of the "screening system" in emergency departments as if it were something new. As detailed in Chapter 1, this plan was in use at the Yale–New Haven Hospital nearly a decade ago. As a result of the success there, it has been adopted in a number of other hospitals. His story is typical of much that has been written for the lay press on this subject, sensational and poorly researched. If lay writers are genuinely interested in bettering the services rendered in hospital emergency departments, they should, before they write, really study the existing problems and seek answers that are constructive and practical. They could only do this by time-consuming observation and, more important, by conferring with knowledgeable people. Observation alone is not enough, for all too often they do not understand what they observe. This subject is too complex and entirely too important to be handled by writers who pose as health authorities one week, legal sages the next, and at other times write on education, religion, or politics.

Q: Are there any national organizations concerned with improvement of emergency department services?

A: Yes. Of course, the American Hospital Association is, but there are others that have worked more specifically in this field. Both the Committee on Trauma of the American College of Surgeons and the American Association for the Surgery of Trauma have long records of interest in this subject. Chapter 19, "Emergency Department Surveys," tells of some of the activity of the Committee on Trauma. More recently, two other organizations have been formed and have functioned long enough to justify their existence. They are (1) the American College of Emergency Physicians, which was organized in September 1968 and is located at 241 East Saginaw Street, East Lansing, Michigan, 48823; and (2) the University Association for Emergency Medical Services, an organization of doctors staffing emergency departments in university connected hospitals, which was organized in October 1969.

Care must be taken that concerned interest in this field does not become diluted by too many organizations. This has happened in other fields of medicine. It is particularly important that a "town and gown" situation be avoided. One way to avoid this is to remember that the primary function of a hospital emergency department is patient care. Research and teaching can be carried out there, and should be, as discussed in Chapter 18, "The Emergency Department as an Educational Center," but they should be secondary to patient service. This is in no way a reflection on the fine trauma research centers that have been organized in a few teaching institutions. They need not detract from the program of immediate, high-grade emergency care.

Some interesting papers read at the meeting of the University Association for Emergency Medical Services at Denver, Colorado, in November 1970 are published in the *Journal of Trauma,* vol. 11, No. 7, July 1971.

Q: *Are there sound arguments against use of interns and residents in emergency departments? Is emergency department service valuable in the training of interns and residents?*

A: The only valid argument against using interns and residents in the care of patients in emergency departments is that it is a bad practice if they are not carefully supervised. This subject has been discussed in some detail in Chapter 7 on staffing and Chapter 18 on the emergency department as an educational center. If the purpose of intern and residency training is to prepare doctors to be of greatest service to their communities, this training (properly supervised) is obviously valuable. It is difficult to agree with Maraveleas and Maraveleas,[2] who state that use of house staff in the emergency department "could jeopardize the entire training program." This attitude represents a narrow view, implying that a physician should learn nothing outside the narrow specialty in which he plans to practice. They say, "Resident rotation through a department which provides diversified services would be contrary to the resident's self-limiting training program." A valid criticism of many specialty training programs is that they are too self-limited. One of the things that has appealed to me about the psychiatric training program that Dr. Branch (see Chapter 17) outlines for his residents is that it includes a period in the emergency department caring for all types of patients. It is valuable for a future psychiatrist to see that people get the outside of their heads split open as well as the inside deranged. It probably would not hurt a gynecologist to know that a kidney might be ruptured or a peptic ulcer perforated. Of course, if the professor of ophthalmology does not want his trainees to be exposed to such things, he should have the right to say so, but I believe the holder of an M.D. degree has some responsibility to the acutely ill or injured patient if he is the only doctor around.

Q: Will the appointment of a group of full-time physicians to staff the emergency department or the letting of a contract to an independent group solve the problems of professional staffing?

A: No. On the contrary, it will increase the problems unless two steps are taken: (1) Restrictions on patient care privileges must be just as stringent as applied to these physicians as to other members of the medical staff. Their training, experience, and ability must be just as thoroughly evaluated as those of attending physicians in the several clinical departments; and (2) The members of the attending staff must be made aware of their responsibilities for cooperative assistance and consultation in the emergency department. Their specialty skills must pick up where those of the emergency department physicians end. It may not be easy to sell this idea to some members of the attending staff, but it must be done. The emergency department physicians must not be looked on as a convenience to relieve the attending physicians when they are off duty or at inconvenient times. The emergency department physicians will, in the course of their normal activities, provide relief for attending physicians, but this is not their primary function.

Q: How may the emergency department physician be protected from being imposed upon?

A: The best solution to this very real danger is to have the group recognized as a full-fledged department of the clinical staff. One of the group should be the director and should have full voting membership on the executive committee, medical board, or whatever term is used in the administrative organization of the medical staff. In the past, emergency departments in some community hospitals have been under the supervision of one of the major clinical departments, most frequently the surgical department. With the increased activity in these departments and the widening scope of their clinical work, they have grown to the point where they deserve departmental status, except in small hospitals, particularly if they have a full-time staff.

Q: *Does the existence of a trauma team or a trauma service alter the need for departmental recognition?*

A: It need not. A trauma team is made up of general and specialty surgeons who take an interest in the care of injured patients. They need not, unless they wish, be involved in the care of all the minor injury cases coming to the department. They can, however, take over the entire responsibility for providing consultation, major emergency accident care, and follow-up care in the more complicated and time-consuming accident cases. There is no standard pattern that need be adhered to in fitting the trauma team into the overall surgical service of the hospital, but where general surgery is subdivided to include, as sections, certain of the surgical specialties, the trauma team may be designated as a section. It must be born in mind that a trauma service is a multidisciplinary service. To make it a subdivision of the orthopedic department or orthopedic service is to fail to recognize that the multiple-injury patient may have problems well beyond the scope of the orthopedist's activities. It is generally, although not unanimously, agreed that a general surgeon with fracture training makes the best leader for a trauma team. Unfortunately, some of our great citadels of surgical training (the current vogue is to call it "education") no longer expose their trainees to the dirty work of caring for accidents. The graduates of these programs may be experts at Whipple procedures or major vascular grafts. They may be able to do transplants that will add a few months or a few years to the life of an already doomed patient, but may not be able to treat a fractured femur or to think of a spinal fracture when the os calcis is smashed in an otherwise healthy person with a long life expectancy. It is to be hoped that if they ever head trauma teams they will know when to call a doctor if they need help.

The idea of trauma teams is a great step forward, and where well organized they have improved the standards of major accident care. However, they are not substitutes for the professional staff of the emergency department, which must include in its round-the-clock activities the entire spectrum of medical and surgical emergencies.

Q: *How can a hospital be sure that a proposed floor plan will be satisfactory to that institution?*

A: The best answer to this important question is to make a life-sized mock-up and go through the motions of patient admission and patient care. Small-scale models are valuable and tell more than architects' drawings, but you can't walk through them; you can only think your way through them. It is surprising that more hospital building committees don't use the life-size mock-up before embarking on what for them is a new concept of construction. A contractor or even the hospital maintenance crew can in a short time, and with few materials other than two-by-fours and ply-wood, lay out enough of the proposed department for trial runs by those who will work in the department. The slight expense will be worthwhile. Don't just look at the layout. Bring in patients on stretchers, register them, put them in the treatment areas, and go through the motions of all neces-sary care. This may show up faulty traffic patterns, awkward location of supplies and equipment, or time-consuming duplications of effort. Study the relationship to other por-tions of the hospital, the direction of door swings, visibility from waiting area into treatment area, and all possible functional features that may come to mind. When this is done, get the committee together and revise the plans. It will be a miracle if no revisions are needed.

Q: *Can and should an emergency department be self-supporting?*

A: First, it *can* with realistic charges for services rendered. A study must be made of all costs, not just those that appear on the surface. There are some hospital costs that involve all departments of the hospital. This goes clear up to administrators' salaries. Any such expenses for services that are not income producing may rightly be spread across the board. However, in budgeting, care must be taken not to overprice certain services. It should be possible at any time to explain and justify any segments of the charges. This will seldom be required, but when a customer buys a high-priced product, he has a right to know why the price is high. Whether the department *should* be self-supporting will depend on the type of hospital, its location, its philosophy, and its administrative guidelines. Chapter 12, "Costs and Fees," discusses this question in more detail.

Q: *How can it be made clear to patients that they owe a doctor's bill and a hospital bill?*

A: This will not be easy in some cases but usually because the patient does not want to understand it rather than that he cannot. The two best guards against misunderstanding on this are an easily read and understood sign in the waiting area and an information brochure stating the policies with regard to the department. It is seldom the patient who really needs the department who complains of the charges. It is usually the one who uses it as a convenience for minor things and then is surprised that the hospital and doctors have taken his case seriously. This is the same patient, who if he is turned away because he doesn't need emergency care, will also complain.

All of the above questions relate to subjects discussed in previous chapters of this book. They were selected for presentation here, because they all refer to problems which seem to have come up in the minds of many hospital people. Of course, hundreds of other questions have been asked, but it is to be hoped that readers will find answers to most of them in the various chapters.

REFERENCES

1. Curing the Emergency Room. *Time,* 98:21, 1971, pp. 94–95.
2. Maraveleas, P.J., and Maraveleas, M.F.: *Emergency Department Group Private Practice.* Troy, Michigan, Medical Ancillary Services, Inc., 1968, p. 3.

Chapter 24

THE LAST WORD

Hospitals planning to build new emergency departments or to reorganize them should seek advice from authoritative sources. Earlier chapters in this book have indicated who may speak with authority. Care must be taken when advisors are sought. There is no substitute for experience. Fancy titles can be misleading. Make sure that your consultants speak from experience, not from theory only.

There are professional hospital consultants who can be of great value in planning, but be wary of the consultant who has a quick answer for every question. Put your faith in one who sometimes doesn't know but is willing to find out. A leading source of knowledge with hospital consultants, as with doctors, is mistakes made previously. In any hospital planning, an experienced architect is essential, but be sure yours is experienced in *hospital* planning. Be more selective than that, be sure that he understands emergency departments. An architectural firm may have a splendid and well-deserved reputation in construction of office buildings and schools but lack the knowledge required for hospital construction. This is a specialty. A careful reading of Chapter 4, "Construction," leaves no doubt that it was written by a specialist. In that chapter there are answers to important questions many trustees, administrators, and doctors would not think to ask.

Valuable as the consultant and architect are, there is no one so valuable as the doctor who has worked in emergency departments and who has had the opportunity to share experiences with other emergency department doctors. If he has also gone through the experience of reorganizing a department and planning new construction, his advice will be doubly valuable. I am surprised how often opportunities are lost because peo-

ple are not willing to visit other places. One of the greatest
rewards of the Emergency Department Survey Program which
has been going on in New Jersey for 15 years has been the
education of those who have made the surveys. It would be
difficult for many of us to list all the good things we have
learned when we went for the purpose of pointing out the bad
things. Although I had had years of experience in caring for
patients in hospitals ranging from 35 to 600 beds and had held
responsible positions in connection with their emergency departments, one of the most valuable periods was the two years
that I was administrative director of the emergency department
in a 430-bed hospital. This was an added duty to my main
responsibility as medical director. It gave me the opportunity to
comprehend the important relationship between the emergency
department and other major departments, both clinical and administrative. It confirmed my already held opinion that there
must be complete cooperation and understanding between all
departments. It also confirmed my opinion that, as many experienced authorities have said, there must be a director in the
department. Probably the two most important accomplishments
during those two years were the planning and early construction of a new department and the recognition of this hospital
service as a major department, with a director who had full
membership on the executive committee of the medical staff.
The emergency department ceased to be a stepchild, with no
one having the necessary authority for its effective administration.

The opportunity to bring up for discussion and often to put
into effect ideas in connection with physical layout was also a
valuable and rewarding experience. In a former assignment, I
had had the opportunity to visit dozens of emergency departments all over the United States, and while on vacation or
attending surgical meetings abroad, I had been shown through
these departments in hospitals in several countries. On many
occasions, the staff working there had pointed out what was
wrong as well as what was right. In planning the new department in the 430-bed hospital, the value of cooperation between
an emergency department committee, a capable administrative

staff, an experienced hospital architect, and a knowledgeable hospital consultant was proven time and time again. Let it not be assumed that there were no arguments or that there was always unanimous agreement, but there was a "meeting of the minds," and everyone involved, including clinical departments, radiologists, anesthesiologists, and nursing service, had the opportunity to influence the planning if they presented sound reasoning.

The plans for the new department were not finalized for nearly two years after the first discussions. This hospital had in the last two decades built a new emergency department on two occasions, but there had never been a thorough planning program. The result was that on both occasions, the plans drawn up and accepted resulted in physical layouts that were far from satisfactory and left many people wondering why such errors had been made. Someone had forgotten to ask the people who work there and insist on their contributing their ideas.

The trends in medical practice and hospital service in this country are not going to lessen the importance of the emergency department. In fact they may well increase it. There is a definite trend toward doctors moving their offices into the hospital, and when they do they will not duplicate in their own professional suites the facilities that are provided in the emergency department. This places more and more responsibility on those who plan these departments for the future. They must not be haphazard facilities, poorly planned and poorly administered. They must be capable of assuming the responsibility for high-grade care of all types of emergencies. It is the hope of the author that this book will make that task a little easier.

INDEX